Witchcraft as a Social Diagnosis

Witchcraft as a Social Diagnosis

Traditional Ghanaian Beliefs and Global Health

Roxane Richter
Thomas Flowers
Elias Kifon Bongmba

LEXINGTON BOOKS
Lanham • Boulder • New York • London

Published by Lexington Books
An imprint of The Rowman & Littlefield Publishing Group, Inc.
4501 Forbes Boulevard, Suite 200, Lanham, Maryland 20706
www.rowman.com

Unit A, Whitacre Mews, 26-34 Stannary Street, London SE11 4AB

British Library Cataloguing in Publication Information Available

Library of Congress Cataloging-in-Publication Data
The hardback edition of this book was previously catalogued by the Library of Congress as follows:

Names: Richter, Roxane, author. | Flowers, Thomas, 1955- author. | Bongmba, Elias Kifon, 1953-
    author.
Title: Witchcraft as a social diagnosis : traditional Ghanaian beliefs and global health / Roxane
    Richter, Thomas Flowers, Elias Bongmba.
Description: Lanham : Lexington Books, [2017] | Includes bibliographical references and index.
Identifiers: LCCN 2016050857 (print) | LCCN 2016051579 (ebook) (print) | LCCN 2016051579
    (ebook)
Subjects: | MESH: Witchcraft | Medicine, African Traditional | Global Health | Ghana
Classification: LCC GR880 (print) | LCC GR880 (ebook) | NLM WB 55.A3 | DDC 615.8/809667—
    dc23
LC record available at https://lccn.loc.gov/2016050857

ISBN 9781498523189 (cloth : alk. paper)
ISBN 9781498523202 (pbk. : alk. paper)
ISBN 9781498523196 (electronic)

We would like to dedicate this book to the women of Gnani. As the ancient Baha'I writing so compellingly states: "The world of humanity is possessed of two wings: the male and the female. So long as these two wings are not equivalent in strength, the bird will not fly."

Contents

List of Figures

Preface

Today's African witchcraft is a mercurial mix of the natural—birth, disease, and death—with the supernatural—spells, spirits, and curses. Yet both can combine to form a punitive force that targets the most vulnerable members of society who cannot fight, protect, or provide for themselves. In certain rural African regions, women can be proclaimed a witch for any number of reasons: They were considered too "bewitchingly" beautiful, or they have been "caught" walking about in the moonlight, or some ill-fated circumstances (a child's death or an outbreak of disease) have been supernaturally linked to them . . . or perhaps they have done nothing more than simply grow too old as a widow to be considered useful to their family and/or society. After they have been accused of using witchcraft, they are (with moral impunity) violently beaten, sometimes even killed, and forever cast out of their family and their village—exiled to live in extreme poverty in a designated witches' village—shunned by the children they birthed, and victimized by a society they once strengthened. Each resident "witch" has a harrowing tale to tell of their journey into hell: Their savage beatings, rejection by family and neighbors, punishments and 'proving' trials, poverty, social excommunication, and coerced confinement in a marginalized community. These are the stories, nonetheless, that must be told. As social scientists, healthcare providers, humanitarian activists, researchers, and fellow human beings, we must affect every means possible to cast a penetrating light upon this dark and often mysterious, misjudged, and profoundly disturbing crisis of culture, religion, law, gender-based and structural violence, and human rights abuses.

This exceptional interdisciplinary biosocial, political, medical, and religious manuscript is an examination of one American medical team's five years of work in the remote northeastern "witches" village of Gnani, Ghana, and the ensuing clashes between traditional Ghanaian beliefs and contemporary Western medical sciences. This unique research brings together the medical, humanitarian, gender, and African religious expertise of three notable co-authors: Roxane Richter, Ph.D., E.M.T., a global healthcare provider, and gender/disaster specialist who has provided aid and medical care in 12 nations; Thomas Flowers, D.O., a U.S. board-certified emergency physician with 32 years of advanced trauma and life support experience who has provided medical care in 8 developing nations; and Elias Kifon Bongmba, Ph.D., a native of Cameroon, and professor of religion at Rice University, who has published on African Witchcraft, African Diaspora Religions, and Religion and Health. This unprecedented text draws on over 1,714 patient interventions, over 95 one-on-one in-depth interviews conducted with the condemned village "witches," as well as rare autobiographical insights provided by Alidu Mahama Zakari, a son of the former (now deceased) Gnani chief.

Over the team's five years of humanitarian medical outreach in Gnani, what was disturbing to Richter and Flowers was the number of patients who had been condemned as witches based (ostensibly) on their medical condition. This seemingly 'undiagnosed outrage' was to provide both the cause and the catalyst for this very research. While there were innumerable examples of this, we will highlight three conditions—albinism, epilepsy, and osteomyelitis—to demonstrate how trauma, disease, and illnesses have been socially "diagnosed" as witchcraft, rather than medically diagnosed as a bacterial infection, and genetic and neurological diseases.

These years of humanitarian service exposed the inherent challenges of dissecting a local patient's supernatural understanding of fate, ill will, and traditional witchcraft—apart from modern scientific interpretation of biological pathogens, structural violence, and disease. These constructive firsthand insights will serve to uncover and examine the rural Ghanaian challenges in social power, gender, religion, political tenets, human rights, medical sciences, and humanitarian aid, as well as its many implications for global partners in search of social justice and gender equity.

As with any society, members of this isolated rural Ghanaian populace grapple with the advent of death, disease, and destruction and thus engage a multiplicity of religious, social power, and cultural mechanisms to construct and fashion a "social diagnosis" befitting a local disease or malady. To that end, many rural Ghanaians maintain complex and multifaceted social mechanisms of religious pluralism, superstition, and traditional beliefs to hold citizens accountable for the fateful, or "evil," and injurious events that happen within their communal realms. Conversely, as scholars and experts in biomedical approaches to health (who are concerned with social justice and gender equity), we routinely attribute biological pathogens, bacteria, and germs for diseases; holding hospitals, doctors, and clinics accountable for prudent and proper medical care as we effect a Western biomedical approach to birth, disease, and death.

Although any exact number of condemned "witches" is difficult to determine, the Anti-Witchcraft Allegation Campaign Coalition-Ghana reports there are approximately 29,928 alleged witches in seven witches' camps (with some 13,287 children) all in northern Ghana; reportedly some 99.9 percent of these condemned witches are exclusively women and children (Laary 2015). These rural people primarily in the Northern, Upper East, and Upper West Regions are accused of being the cause of crop failure, illness, impotence, death, or financial misfortune. One very distinctive feature of the Gnani (also spelled as "Nani," or "Ngani," or "N'gani") village is that it is the only "witches" camp in the northern region of Ghana that allows male "witches," known as "wizards." Our approach to this research is to offer a new perspective on witchcraft as we examine the voices of the innumerable people who have been accused, condemned, and sentenced to what many consider a life of marginalized exile, due to disease and illness. Our project also probes questions of abuse, torture, and maltreatment, seeking to extrapolate how diseases, injuries, and illnesses they suffer are related to their social condition, as well as the overarching dialogue and contestation of witchcraft.

From the outset, we do not assume that all Ghanaians have the same view of witchcraft. There are those who continue to see it as a supernatural activity which is a necessary segment of the social fabric, and thus claim that one cannot simply disregard it. Others regard witchcraft as nothing more than activities of anti-social members of society who have chosen to use those capacities for their own private gain(s). Some, on the other hand, think that the rest of the global contemporary society no longer believes in witchcraft and instead follow science and scientific developments, so much so that modern science is often seen as 'Western witchcraft.' Those individuals would be very surprised to follow the literature on witchcraft in the Western world today. Ghanaian scholar of religion, Kofi Asare Opoku, defined witchcraft as the: "employment of esoteric power for a definite purpose, good or evil" (1978, 146). The literature on witchcraft in Ghana emphasizes also that one of the better ways of understanding the phenomenon is to look at it in context of the different forms of misfortune that people experience and the strategies they employ to resolve those issues (Assimeng 1989). In a very broad sense, Ghanaians deem witchcraft as something that one can acquire when they are born if the mother is a witch; witchcraft can also be passed on from one person to another through exchange of material substances of gifts (Opoku 1978). People also believe that witches tend to work together and form guilds or association through which they carry out their intentions (Akrong 2007). Witchcraft accusations have increased in light of growing social problems and economic pressures, particularly citing rises in: seasonal rainy season famines, familial tensions, an increase in women's leisure/free time;

mounting male/patriarchal frustration(s); general insecurity; economic deprivation; food insecurity, and the availability of witchcraft as "an easy solution" to disputes and difficulties (Kirby 2012, 203). As our study will demonstrate, the decline in the state of public health in some regions has accompanied a rise in illnesses (especially through pandemics of Ebola and HIV/AIDS), elevating fears that witches are producing many maladies. Even in this new context, the literature on witchcraft demonstrates that some of the ancient views on witchcraft remain. As examples, witches are still accused of killing a person and consuming that person's flesh, also witchcraft is believed to primarily affect family/kinfolk members. Oftentimes when people experience success in trade or profession, they believe they have succeeded due to witchcraft powers; conversely when they fail, an accusing finger is pointed at someone for (negatively) 'bewitching' them. Therefore there is a general view in society that witches are real and responsible for all the evil things that go on in society (Akrong 2007). Elom Dovlo argues: "powers attributed to 'witches' include the ability to inflict material loss through fire, theft, crop failure, . . . poor spending . . . sterility, impotence or disease such as leprosy" (2007, 68). Witchcraft is blamed for the majority of adversities and misfortunes (Apter 1993).

In this book, we will begin our discourse within the historical context of the study, situating Ghana in the Post-Colonial context and notable national achievements and challenges. We then argue that there is still a strong urban/rural divide in Ghana that has significantly raised the tenor of the discourse, as well as provided some local justification for the concept of and the actual establishment of these witches' villages. Based on research in Ghana, this chapter will discuss the beliefs about witches, their role in society, the alleged power they possess and how they reportedly employ that power. We will also explore the idea of prejudice which makes it possible for others to designate, isolate, and discriminate against others they deem "witches." Preliminary research gives us some indications that we must question why accusations are accepted at "face value"—and sentences of exile pronounced, with no local and/or national authorities exploring alternative methods of addressing these local conflicts. We will discuss these perspectives in dialogue with indigenous beliefs about witchcraft in Ghana and examine some examples from other African communities. Our emphasis will be on local perspectives in the community of the research and the members of the witches' village of Gnani. While there is a robust discussion of witchcraft in Ghana from the past, recent studies have discussed the concerns about the practice largely in light of Pentecostal beliefs and churches in Ghana. Some of these studies have offered a sustained theological critique from the Pentecostal tradition (Meyer 2012). Popular culture has also taken up the theme of witchcraft in Ghana (Meyer and Pels 2003). The virtue of these studies is the manner in which they demonstrate contemporary concerns, fascinations with witchcraft, and document the use of spiritual resources to combat these beliefs. Thus we will conclude the chapter by placing the discussion and analyses of the interviews in the context of religious multiplicity in the region, focusing briefly on Islamic, Christian, and African traditional religious perspectives on witches and the practice of witchcraft.

In the second chapter we will discuss in expansive terms what day-to-day life is like in one of the witches' villages, based on our years of research in the village of Gnani in the Yendi municipality in northern Ghana. The history of the region, which has progressed through many years of violence, will begin with the inter-ethnic violence in 1980, and follow its history through the ensuing political and indigenous instabilities. This chapter also looks at how this small community—constructed on stigma—has become a communal residence for the socially condemned. The "voices of the women" will be heard in several of the 95 one-on-one interview sessions conducted in 2008 and 2015. Multifaceted processes and traditional practices concerning the accusation, transport, judgement, and conviction of accused witches will also be outlined and defined.

In chapter 3, we will place witchcraft in a broader context when we examine biological mechanisms and medical concepts of disease and illness, introducing biomedical concepts in attempts to further examine local Ghanaian, African, and Western etiologies of disease. We will begin this by exploring modern-day scientific enquiries into some possible physiological causes for historical witchcraft accusations during the American witch trials in Salem, Massachusetts, between 1692 and 1693. We will then expand this situational context by examining the states of urban and rural health systems to understand the two paradigms of healing, access, and capabilities to treat illnesses and diseases in contemporary Ghana. What follows will be a contemporary discourse of endemic diseases—and their probable associations to witchcraft indictments—such as: communicable diseases (HIV/AIDS, TB, and Leprosy); malaria; epilepsy and seizures; albinism; mental illnesses; the curse of multiple births; and vision care challenges.

In the fourth chapter, our hypothesis is that some demonstrable clinical medical identification(s) in our 1,714 patient records may be one key to understanding some of these illnesses, in that a proper diagnosis by a skilled healthcare provider could alleviate some of the misconceptions that have led to witchcraft accusations. It is in this context that we also explore some of the health conditions, injuries, and illnesses that have been witnessed and treated at our "Clinics without Walls." The most common and endemic diseases we have observed are communicable diseases such as HIV/AIDS, malaria, epilepsy, parasites, malnutrition, bacterial and viral infections, albinism, and possible mental health issues. We will also discuss our findings in the context of an analysis of etiology of diseases and disorders which fuel accusations and encourage the "blame game." Given the unique medical data that we are generating, we will conclude our data analyses by reviewing the medical findings and how they relate to witchcraft accusations, livelihood opportunities, chronic diseases, gender-disaggregated evidence(s), and more. At the chapter's conclusion, we will also cite some of our most memorable on-the-ground challenges and notable "lessons learned" when offering our provisional cross-cultural medical care.

Our fifth chapter will examine pathologies of prejudice employed via social mechanisms. At its genesis, we will delve into structural violence as a controlling social mechanism. Here we will approach the discourse from a social justice and human rights perspective, institutionalized violence, and gender-based violence as it is informed by feminist theory. A feminist research epistemology was employed in this research since feminism's most engaging and persuasive epistemological insight is deemed by noted feminist scholars (Doucet and Mauthner 2006, and Lennon and Whitford 1994) as the conjoining of constructs of knowledge and power. We will therefore critically examine witchcraft as a feminist discourse that imposes prejudice, misogyny, patriarchal control, and discrimination. However, this linear discourse will be broadened to encompass violence and abuse against elderly women, "the world's fastest growing demographic group" which includes "sexual violence, property grabbing, financial abuse, and increasingly, extreme violence against older women accused of witchcraft," according to a 2014 United Nations report (1). Therefore the structural violence evident in an elderly female widow's or "witch's" poor quality of life—including acute hypertension from (due to stressful environs), poor vision (due to no optometry treatment access) and blindness from untreated cataracts, crippling osteoarthritis, and other illnesses that typically befall any elderly person who works hard physical labor with insufficient access to nourishing food, or medical, dental, or eye care—will be detailed.

Our last chapter will delve into the dialectics and dynamics of witchcraft in contemporary Ghanaian society, and address how the current national media content serves to eradicate, indoctrinate, or cultivate witchcraft beliefs via TV, radio, homegrown "Kumawood," and Nigerian "Nollywood" films, as well as voluminous social media mechanisms. While precise data would be problematic to ascertain, recent studies show that "about 90 percent of Ghanaians believe in witches and in witchcraft" (Dunn 2015, 1). It is in this final review that we will also consider legal, constitutional, and human rights perspectives that call for legal intervention, enforcement, and prosecution of discrimination against people on the suspicion that there are witches. We will address the quandaries of contemporary lawmakers, police, human rights activists, and members of the legal profession (who have in the past attempted to regulate, investigate, and/or enforce litigation and/or criminal penalties for the unmerited prosecution of witches) who face questionable testimonies, dubious circumstantial evidence, and arbitrary accusations. We will conclude the book by addressing the implications of our findings, and offering ten recommendations that each draw from our research, medical data, and examination of the spiritual, medical, and economic conditions of the Gnani residents. These 10 abridged recommendations are placed together in a succinct listing in order to streamline the reader's enumeration of the recommendations; the discourse, defense, justifications, and supporting evidence(s) can be found in research's associated topics and aforementioned chapters.

This research is not concerned with new forms of witchcraft per se, but we are interested in pursuing the social stigma and segmentation which has found a unique expression in the notion and reality of one witches' village, Gnani, in northern Ghana. What we also bring to this discourse that is original is the perspective of American medical professionals who will share their contrasting stories of scientifically diagnosed diseases and illnesses—such as seizures, tuberculosis, albinism, HIV/AIDS, and malaria—in striking contrast with views that perceive these patients as powerful sorcerers and witches. These medical discussions will follow due protocol and respect the privacy of patients, and where consent was given, we will share photographs that give insights into the social world and the medical conditions which many people in the witches' village endure. We will examine the exile imposed on these women and the few men in our area of study, and raise questions from a comparative perspective about the reliability of this manner of solution to witchcraft accusation. Using data from five years of medical work, 1,714 patient records, and 95 one-on-one interviews, we will propose new approaches and offer policy proposals that could generate a conversation on witchcraft in contemporary society that would reject exile as a viable and judicious solution.

This research's target audiences include scholars in African studies, healthcare professionals, scholars of global health and emergency medicine, students of all academic levels, as well as individuals, nonprofits/nongovernmental organizations (NGOs), and organizations interested in the current trends in global healthcare challenges. We also bring a novel theoretical perspective which will include other academics and scholars engaging in interdisciplinary research in African studies, religion, and studies of magic, witchcraft, and the occult. We are convinced that the issues raised in this interdisciplinary study will be relevant to a number of individuals as well as numerous gender, human rights/social justice, religion, rural and urban, global healthcare, jurisprudence, cross-cultural, multicultural, and/or African Studies research.

In the end, the goal of this research is not to resolve whether or not these witchcraft accusations and claims are indeed accurate. Witchcraft accusations reflect a social view of the world that has endured many centuries. Thus we are principally interested in mapping the new social dynamics which characterize contemporary understandings of witchcraft. We will focus particularly on the gender, human rights, structural violence, and medical (etiologies of illness and diseases) dimensions of witchcraft. To do this, we will document the personal stories and accounts of witchcraft accusations labeled against the "witches," the stigma, isolation, and discrimination they have experienced, as well as the disease and illness issues they have encountered—which are presumed to be either their justified fate, or integrated into the current witchcraft discourse.

Acknowledgments

Throughout the years of our rural medical outreaches, we have had many generous donors, hospitals, pharmaceutical companies, medical equipment and supply manufacturers, and volunteers to thank. We are greatly indebted to honorable Kofi Nsiah Poku and Kina Pharma for their immeasurable generosity in supporting our medical outreaches in Ghana. We want to thank other generous donors, volunteers, and benevolent support from: Dr. Salifu Bawa (Central Regional Hospital, Cape Coast), Ghana; Gifty Mante, RN (God's Gift Maternity Clinic, Ekumfi, Ghana); Dr. Didier Amehi; Sophie Mawussi Adahji; Dr. Charles Darko-Takyi (Professor of the University of Cape Coast, Ghana, School of Optometry and his many graduate student volunteers); Ethicon; Johnson & Johnson; W.T. Cutts and American Tank & Vessel; Stephen Jones and Clear Lake Regional Hospital Medical Staff; Crystal Crafters and Dr. Tom Pruett (optometrist); Jerry Higgins (optician); Most Rev. Eric Doku of the Ghana Methodist Church; Alidu Mahama Zakari of Yendi, Ghana; Herzstein Foundation; Heart to Heart International/MAP International nonprofit and Merck Pharmaceuticals (for low-cost and at-cost prescription medications, supplies, and hospital-grade equipment); Greater Houston Emergency Physicians; CeraLyte oral rehydration products; Christus St. John's Hospital; Abbott Laboratories; Clear Lake United Methodist Church's youth group; Slade Lewis and Lewis Jewelers; MODEC Inc.; and many, many others throughout the years. We also want to personally thank Bishop Joseph Atto Brown and his (now-deceased) wife Maud Brown, who were our favorite Ghanaian smiles, warmest "*Akwaaba*" ("You are welcome") in-country hosts, and our selfless co-laborers in the field. I should also comment on the congenial relationship with my chief, Nana Kwefi Arkoh, of Ekotsi-Bogyano. And last but not least, one very special thanks goes out to our dear friends and co-laborers, Jack and Diane Webb, who serve as U.S. Honorary Consul General to Ghana in Houston, Texas. Throughout the years, Jack and Diane have supported our teams with travel visas, donations, capacity and relationship building, and ever since our first ventures out to Ghana, they have become our stalwart 'backbone' of our in-country organizational support.

Research Assistance: We are indebted to our three primary research assistants, including: Rainier W. Richter, Christian Lovins, and Alidu Zakari. Our Texas-based assistants, Rainier W. Richter and Christian Lovins served as our astute data analysts and statisticians for this project. Our Ghana-based assistant, Alidu Zakari, served not only as our translator in Ghana but also assisted us in conducting all of our one-on-one interview sessions, and in providing historical and folk knowledge concerning the Gnani village and its people.

Chapter One

History, Tradition, and Religion

Witchcraft studies in Africa went through a renaissance in the last three decades with research and publications, which could arguably be said, that have barely caught up with the depth and gravity of the belief in witchcraft in many communities. Yet the new studies, which have grown exponentially, have expanded the vocabulary and demonstrated the malleability of the concept of witchcraft. The new studies are marked by a continuity and discontinuity. The continuity is reflected in the very idea of witchcraft, which is conceptualized as a power that others claim can be acquired or inherited and used for both good and evil. However, many who suspect or think that they are victims of the negative use of such supernatural powers interpret witchcraft as a negative force and therefore oppose any such beliefs and alleged practices. They do so because they think that such powers are deployed to cause misfortune to a person or a community (Evans-Pritchard 1937; Douglas 1970). Communities have engaged in witch-finding activities for decades as a way of detecting and punishing witches (McLeod 1957; Auslander 1993). The fixation and tenacity with which communities have pursued witchcraft and its alleged practitioners demonstrates that witchcraft is tied to ideas concerning morality, the "common good," and welfare in many communities (Crick 1970; Bongmba 2001).

Many of the witchcraft accusations are leveled against relatives or people with whom the accused person supposedly has some connection (Bongmba 2001). In the past, once a community had gone through the process of identifying, accusing, or extracting confessions from alleged witches, severe sanctions were meted out. In many cases such sanctions involved trials, beatings, punishments, banishment into exile, and/or death (as in the cases of the Gnani women involved in this study). Witchcraft has remained an ambivalent concept, considered dangerous, yet it continues to draw interest from

1

Africans, Muslims, and Christians. In this twenty-first century, people are still forced to drink potions ("medicines" with unknown and potentially harmful and/or toxic ingredients) to prove their innocence. In 2009, Amnesty International reported that President Yahyah Jamneh of Gambia ordered that 1,000 people suspected of practicing witchcraft be arrested and forced to drink a hallucinogenic substance as a way of controlling witchcraft in the country. It was reported that witch-hunters traveled from village to village accompanied by Gambian security forces, underscoring the evident state sanctioning of this misguided approach to witchcraft eradication.

The discontinuity in the studies of witchcraft is marked by a number of issues that are best summed up by the expression "modernity"—a problematic notion which is difficult to define as it is not restricted to a historical understanding of the term "modern" in terms of what some consider the modern period. Accordingly, most studies of witchcraft in Africa would be categorized as "modern" (Geschiere 1997). But the term makes sense in the study of witchcraft, if one understands it as beliefs and activities that occur within contemporary society and continue to defy scientific evidence; or in the case religious interpretations, a failure to take into account developments in textual and contextual interpretations. In this regard, witchcraft is a quintessential problematic issue of "modernity" as it is open (or applied) to contemporary issues in manners that are compelling both to those who affirm that witchcraft is powerful and effective, and critics who see no role for witchcraft today (Fisiy and Rawlands 1989). Recent studies demonstrate that witchcraft is no longer a phenomenon that takes place in small villages, rather an urban phenomenon, including all the manipulations of the "normal," and affecting power relations in postcolonial societies where people are grappling with the vicissitudes of a global economy (Ashforth 1998; Ardener 1970; Niehaus 2001; Pels1998). If modernity has been infected by witchcraft or vice versa—one thing is clear: This new twist to a perennial social logic has infected all vectors of social life (Geschiere 1997; Lyons 1998; Schmoll 1993; Mburu 1979; Mpolo 1976; 1975). One clear difference in studies and analyses of witchcraft in scholarship is the expansion of vocabulary as scholars increasingly use local terms to distinguish between a broad world of ideas and practices signified by the English term "witchcraft" (Bongmba 1998; Bokie 1993). One of the most interesting modern twists to understanding witchcraft remains the religious dimension and the diabolical interpretations that offer the new religious powers to exorcise and cast out witchcraft (Meyer 1991; 1999). Our study reflects the dialectics of the historical and contemporary discourses of witchcraft and we focus on the accusations leveled against women who then were exiled to live in witch's village.

HISTORICAL VIEWS ON INDIGENOUS AFRICAN WITCHCRAFT

Witchcraft accusations have been documented in Ghana for a long time. Contrary to the research studies published by Meyer Fortes and later by Margaret Field (whose 1939 study argued that witchcraft was not a major pre-occupation in the northern territories) but that the northern region had a reputation for having "strong medicine" that could control witchcraft (Fortes 1949; Field 1940). The situation led some people in the region to travel to the Northern Territories to find protective medicines where it was thought the deities of the region specialized in witchcraft (Field 1940).

Nonetheless, David Tait published two studies on sorcery in the region that are germane to understanding present day witchcraft discourses and practices in the Gnani area. In his essay, "Konkomba Sorcery," Tait pointed out that the relevant terms of *osũo* (pl. *besuom*) and the class of sorcerers was designated as *kasuo*, referred to 'evil' in general (Tait 1954). It is important to point out here that Tait used sorcery to refer to the use of 'medicines' to kill someone. In that sense it differs from witchcraft that we see in the region today, but the hunt of individuals for using such medicines bears some resemblances to witchcraft accusations. As Tait himself would note in later essays, the 'medicines' that were used in the region were said to be connected to shrines that existed in the south and were transferred to the northern areas of Ghana in colonial times. In Konkomba society, the "medicines" were simply called "sorcerer's medicines." Tait also referred to the notion of *transvection* as behavior which refers to notions that sorcerers fly about at night to attack and harm other people, something that is linked to witchcraft in various regions of Ghana and other African regions.

While we do not claim that the discourses and institutions associated with witchcraft in present day descend from these studies, Tait's analysis provide broad insights into what could have been the genesis of what we see in Gnani today. Tait's later study, "A Sorcery Hunt in Dogomba," clearly demonstrates a strong antecedent to what we see in northern Ghana today (1963). In that 1963 study we learn that in Konkomba society sorcerers kill their victims by incarnating into a snake and waylaying the victim. The second method involved sending a shadow of the sorcerer to eat the shadow of the victim, causing the death of the victim through a lingering disease. When witchcraft 'medicines' were used exclusively, they would be placed in a drink, in kola nuts, or along a path where the victim would pass. In these instances it was believed that sorcerers hid the poison in their thumbnails, and discreetly transferred them into the substances that would be consumed by others. People therefore kept their fingernails closely trimmed. In cases of *transvection*, entrances into compounds were shut at night and no one slept alone, except single women (without children)—and nighttime visitors were forced to loudly announce their presence, or risk being beaten with flaming sticks. If someone feared that they could become a victim of an attack, that person took medicines called *idabin* to defend themselves. If an individual waited too long, and the attack had already been implemented, it was considered too late, and there was nothing that would ward off the impending spell.

Tait also argued that close agnatic (patrilineal) relatives can be accused of being sorcerers, but in order to do so, one would have to wait and see if an illness worsens, or some calamitous event occurred. In the Konkomba society, men are also accused of being witches. Therefore anyone in the society can be accused of sorcery (Tait 1954). Sorcery can be transmitted from parent to child, through teaching. At the time of the study, Tait reported that sorcerers were no longer being killed, but women were still running away to safe havens after being accused. The differences between male and female treatment was indicated by Tait's claim that men moved only when they have been repeatedly accused, and then only moved back to their place of birth or a new section of the region.

It was believed in the area that when a sorcerer died, his medicines died with him, and the Tallensi also claim that witchcraft could be transmitted through kin descent, breaching the notion that "medicines" could also be transferred through generations. In the Dagomba study, we learn that the Nantonlana of Savelugu invited a specialist to carry out a hunt as villagers had seen a "sorcerer's fire" in the night. Tait noted that the flashing fire traveled about 30 or 40 feet above the ground, noting: "It may be a large firefly, though it does not resemble any firefly I have seen close to. In Kokomba country I thought (though I never say it there) that it might be an effect of marsh gas," and the first news of the movement was in July of 1955 in Savelugu, and "then the first phase of it in Nanton" (Tait 1963, 136). Tait reported that the witch hunt had three phases: First accusations were made against the so-called sorcerers. In the village of Nyemando, a man and five women had gone to a shrine *bugele* also called *Nana* located in Gefsiego. The man's mother was accused of sorcery. Five other women and their husbands (from same family) were also accused of sorcery. The man stayed at the shrine for five days and drank the "medicine" which made him see other sorcerers. In the village of Nanton, all the women were told to gather in front of the chief's house and the seers danced among the women to detect the sorcerers. The women who were not accused were asked to stand before the chief, and some were accused. The accused then went and drank the medicines that would destroy the "medicine" of the sorcery at Guſeigo and Karaga. The process took about three days—and out of fifty women, only one was accused of being a sorcerer. The women drank two kinds of "medicines": the first one was to determine if a person was a sorcerer, and the second kind of "medicine" enabled a non-sorcerer see what other sorcerers were doing. Among the Wimbum of the Northwest Province in Cameroon, this secondary type of "medicine" would be the substances that are given to a "non-witch" to enable them to have *tʉ yebu* ("to see things"). In Dagomba society, the women who were accused were asked to release the souls of the persons they had held captive and were getting ready to kill. The women "released" their victims by washing them in yet another "medicine."

The terms for sorcerer in Dagbane is "*pagkurugu*" and refers to both male and female sorcerers, but the term "*pagjura*" refers to only female sorcerers, as the majority of the accused were women (Tait 1963). What is important for us to note here is that Tait reported that after this hunt, things returned to normal, and the women who were accused were welcome to remain in their familial homes. Therefore forced exile is not a general practice in the northern region, nor among the Dagomba, but places of refuge, and prior tests/ treatments formerly existed in the region. There was no violence during the first phase Tait recorded, as the district clerk of the local council warned people that violence would not be tolerated. In the Dagomba context, most of the accusations involved members of the household. Tait argued at the time:

> It is said in Dagomba that the person most feared is the father's sister, either as a sorcerer herself or as one who, if her own father be dead, has direct access to the ancestors and may therefore remove the ritual protection of the ancestors from a victim in the same descent group. (Tait 1963, 136)

Since there is no widow's inheritance in that society, if a woman's husband dies, she returns to her parents' home. It explains why in some of the interviews the women said that they had returned to live in their father's compound after the death of their husbands. It is for this reason that some of the women in the interviews said that they were living in their father's household when the accusations against them were made. In the Konkomba areas, accusations were made along clan lines, and hence victims were not always members of the household.

What was clear in Tait's analysis is that in the first of the three phases most of the accusations were women accusing other women, and age did not seem to be a barrier to the accusations. In the second and third phases, some of the accusers had junior status within the household, and most of the accusers were married women (primarily senior wives wielding powerful statuses). While he did not know the social status of all the women in the first phase, Tait pointed out that the majority of the women in the second and third phase were married to prominent men, and most of the Dagomba victims, or accusers, were Muslims. In further analyses of the third phase, Tait indicated that a woman admitted to killing two sons of a rich neighbor. One woman denied the accusations even though she was roughly handled. One woman was told she had killed her grandson; however she did not deny it. One woman admitted to killing a young relative. Another woman said she did not know the person she was accused of killing and she was told it was her husband's younger brother. And yet another woman was accused of killing the son of her brother, in whose house she was living after the birth of her child. Tait found out that the victims were mostly young males, something that could reinforce the gender dimension of witchcraft accusations. Since primarily women are accused, they are targeted and accused of bringing misfortunes that chiefly affect young males (who toil on farms). During this time of great stress, as the crops were failing, the younger women were accusing the older women and widows, who may not be as dependent on the down-turn in production. But Tait suspected that the increase may also have been motivated by the prevalence of cheap new medicine that was supposed to detect/protect from witchcraft through the cult of Nana. As to the hunt, Tait pointed out that it seemed primarily as an opportunity to vent frustrations and personal animosity against others. The members of the society were traumatized, even if they were not directly accused. The *Tindana* in Tamale thought that these medicines were introduced to the region recently, but Tait notes that the issues had very much to do with socially approved use of magic and medicines.

The account first given by David Tait did not indicate if the participants tried to state their innocence, but it was clear that the people believed that there were witches all over and something had to be done. While the Nana cult did not leave a lasting impact on the region, one could argue that what would develop later followed their earlier movements, as John Parker found that a major problem in the *Talensi* area was *soob* (witches), bringing many people to the Tongnaab shrines (Parker 2006). Parker argues, rightly in our opinion, that while one has not taken time to compare the historical record and the discourses on witchcraft today, there is no doubt in the minds of some people that witches are believed to hurt people in contemporary Ghana, especially in the north where rituals related to witchcraft eradication abound. John Parker has argued that the northern regions of Ghana were believed to have potent medicines and rituals that were employed in the south in witch-finding (Parker 2006). Witchcraft in the region shared many of the same characteristics (as other parts of the country), and were said to possess the power to consume the souls of other people, causing them to die. Witches could also fly at night, and had doubles (*doppelgangers*), and they possessed the power to transform into those doubles (Parker 2006). It was believed that people transformed into their doubles and roamed around at night in the region, a belief that is widespread in West and Central Africa. In Cameroon, many stories are told about an animal that was shot, and the animal—before taking its last breath—reincarnates back into the person whose life they have "possessed," confesses their evil crime, and dies. In the northern territories these stories did not generate anti-witchcraft movements as the south had seen in colonial times. We are interested in the account Parker gives as he discusses the practice of Nana (a southern title) a healing cult in 1955, when women traveled to the Gusheigu District in the Dagbon area, hence the idea having been transplanted from the southern region (Parker 2006).

WITCHCRAFT AND THE EXIGENCIES OF TEMPORALITY

When a person visits Gnani for the first time, one of the questions one might ask is when will these women go home? The houses in which they live are small, and they have very little by way of personal belongings. Each resident has a bed, space for their clothes and other belongings, a hearth where she can cook inside the house if it rains, and she cannot cook outside, plus some storage space for food. Each person also has a small granary outside their hut where they store food for the season. The signs of temporality are present everywhere in the village. The location—its distance from the main village, the youthful and sparse vegetation, and the few domesticated animals—all reveal the temporality of existence in this witches' village. One could argue that life in many respects (even from a cultural and symbolic perspective) reflects temporality. Yet the structures and institutions humans dream, imagine, and construct often express a yearning for permanence. The sense of permanence is reinforced by notions like nationality, region, ethnicity, village, and quarters within villages. These demarcations, even in modern pluralistic nations of Africa or other parts of the world, point to a human desire for a sense of rootedness and means of managing temporality, even though these social and communal settings and structures spell permanence and a sense of home.

However, there are times when we, as human beings, are compelled to invoke and embrace the temporal, as with the residents of Gnani. The leader of the Gnani women said that she was brought to the village on the advice of her brother, as she was accused of using witchcraft to cause the illness of her nephew. At the time the accusation was made, she was living with her brother, as her husband had died. When she was accused, she expected her brother and relatives to speak on her behalf, but neither her brother nor any of her other relatives did so. Instead he advised her to come to the village and drink the medicines that would detect witchcraft, but also remove any witchcraft power she might have possessed. When she came to the village, she decided to live there for the rest of her life, even though she was found to be innocent. However the 'medicine' she drank was also used to "purify" and "protect" her in the village.

The irony is that what might have been thought of as a temporal sojourn has morphed into a permanent residence. Most of the residents of Gnani stated emphatically that they did not want to return or be repatriated back to their home villages. They had been falsely accused, forced to leave their families and homes, so many of the women were adrift in "no man's land."

They realized that the fearful climate concerning witchcraft in the region made it difficult for members of their families to openly support them. In many cases, family members were the accusers who pressed the charges, telling them to go to the witches' village. They were betrayed by their families and their communities and they did not see any reason to go back. Some say if they did not leave they would have been subjected violence. Therefore even after being in the witches' village for many years—they still fear for their very lives. Speaking from their experience in the witches' village, many of them have also said that they do not want to go back to their respective homes. Many of them are longtime residents of Gnani, and Gnani is home.

For instance, "Grace" was asked if she would return to her father's compound since she had been exonerated. She stated emphatically that she wanted to die in the witches' village. She had been sent to the village accused of being responsible for two deaths, her son and her husband. "Grace" had six children, and two miscarriages, and all died. Her father asked her to go to the witches' village for her own safety. Since then, he had also passed away, so "Grace" thought there was no way for her to return now. The village was a place of peace for her and she did not see any reason to disrupt her life by going back to her own village.

To understand these dynamics, we must consider some of the rather unique aspects of the village's processes. When a person is brought to the village, the priest carries out a divination to determine if the person is a witch. As with most of the residents, they indicated that they were exonerated. Yet regardless of the divination's verdict, the priest administers "medicines" that will (supposedly) treat the desire and power to engage in witchcraft. Here we should note the symbolism associated with these actions; the medicines do not seek to accuse, curse, or exile, but rather act as a comfort, assurance, and sign of integration into a new community—a powerful and empowering notion for someone who is now feared as "dangerous" and evil. We think that this welcoming introduction into the community is at the heart of the experiences of the many members of the community. The residents talk of having peace. They do not live in fear anymore. They have established relationships in the village and do not see any reason why they should disrupt those relationships. One woman indicated that she could go back to her children, but not to her husband's home where they had falsely accused and exiled her.

From our own experience and work in the region, an important contributor to such action would be to rethink the challenges these regions face in education and public health, one of the recommendations of ActionAID, a nonprofit organization that has worked in the area. While we recognize that belief in witchcraft is rooted in the world view of the people, it is also clear from some of the interviews conducted with the residents of the village in Gnani that the residents are aware that some of the deaths for which they were accused and exiled for decades resulted from untreated, treatable medical conditions. While witchcraft exists in Ghana and many other regions in Africa, our records indicate that the public health needs of the region far outweigh most of the regions in Ghana. Any steps taken to address the social world in which beliefs like witchcraft thrives cannot ignore public health. We explore these issues in the next sections of the book.

RELIGIOUS MULTIPLICITIES: ISLAM, CHRISTIANITY, AND AFRICAN TRADITIONAL BELIEFS

From our personal and professional interactions and observations, Ghana is a deeply religious nation. It is estimated that 71.2 percent of the population is Christian (including a growing Pentecostal community) that makes up about 28.3 percent, and a minority Muslim population comprising about 17.6 percent who primarily reside in the Northern Region. About 5.2 percent of the Ghanaian population practice traditional religion, and religion and spirituality play important roles in the daily lives of people. Christianity has made great gains since the last decades of the twentieth century through the explosive growth of Pentecostalism (Gifford 2004). Accounts of witchcraft involve local religions, and other traditional religions such as Christianity and Islam. Members of religious communities still express strong beliefs and take measures to protect themselves. The growing business of exorcism among Christian leaders demonstrates the strong beliefs in witchcraft in Ghana. There are shrines in the south and the north that have been consulted to address the issues of witchcraft. While religious communities may have differences, and Christians, especially Pentecostals, tend to see traditional religion as irrelevant, with many considering witchcraft a contemporary conundrum.

Historically, there is a strong affinity between religion and witchcraft in the village of Gnani—where religion plays a pivotal purpose in the lives of the members of the community. Traditional religion is practiced both among the Dagomba and Konkomba. They both believe in a "Supreme Being" who is the creator of the world. The earth is regarded with great respect especially among the Konkomba, who refer to the Earth divinity as *Kiting,* and *Kitalangban* is a heavenly deity who is responsible for keeping the earth fertile (Zimon 2003). The earth divinity *Kiting,* is the parent of Uwumbor. Henryk Zimon has pointed out that "the earth is the divinity, spirit, the source of life principles, fertility, well-being, and richness" (2003, 422). There are indications then that the Konkomba see the earth as a divine being that connects them with their ancestors and their land. The priest *utindaan* occupies an important place in the lives of the people and is often referred to as the "owner" of the land. The priest and the chief cannot come from the same lineage. After the priest has been chosen by the "Earth Spirit," he is then installed in his office, where he has shrine to carry out his religious rituals. He keeps the religious traditions alive and upholds moral imperatives in the community, including prohibition of murder, adultery, and incest "pollute" the earth. In the past those who committed these violations suffered harsh consequences such as drought or infertility, and were punished by expulsion or death. The priest works closely with elders of the community to settle discord and disagreements within the community. Yet perhaps his most important function is to diagnose the source of misfortune and to offer solutions such as the establishment of the witches' village.

This special responsibility of the priest in the Konkomba community is similar to the responsibilities of the priest in the Gnani witches' village. He is a diviner who determines the causes and sources of misfortune. Recent literature, especially on the witches' village, tends to describe the priest as a "fetish priest." We had heard the term used by several Ghanaian evangelical pastors and local clergy. During one of our visits, people from a surrounding village came to consult the local priest about a death in their community. We were asked for a token gift for observing the ceremony, but the local minister admonished us for wasting our money by giving it to a fetish priest. This exchange reminded us of the challenges traditional religions have had in Ghana and in other parts of Africa. In colonial Ghana, traditional rites were treated in various ways. Natasha Gray has argued that colonial governments tried to curb traditional religious rites in an attempt to "protect the public from 'superstition,'" and allow colonial officials to ban sects that encouraged those practices (in efforts to frustrate any attempts by people to seek the assistance of their local gods) (Gray 2005). Nonetheless, these efforts did not deter people from seeking these local religious remedies as many of the local anti-witchcraft activities continued. As Gray points out:

> The tenacity of belief in outlawed gods is an unexplored aspect of the religious life of colonial Ghana that that has important historical implications. Periodic discoveries of the Akan public's belief that their gods were independent of the dictates of colonial law contributed to the government's slow realization that attempts to discredit traditional religion exposed the weaknesses of the state more than the gods. (2005, 139)

While we must be cautious about generalizing, especially since Gray writes about southern Ghana, however what Gray says about the outcome of the colonial state's interventions in traditional religion is important in light of the things that take place in villages like Gnani for three reasons. First, some people in Ghanaian communities still regard traditional religious beliefs as efficacious, and therefore there is still a strong commitment to traditional religious beliefs—causing members of different communities turn to those religious ideas in time of crisis. We should add that this is not a rejection of either Christianity or Islam, but merely the practice of a religious bricolage that has worked for many people in Ghana and other parts of Africa. Secondly, Gray is correct that the reality of local religious beliefs in the face of colonial attempts to dismantle some of its practices failed because when the public perceived a crisis, proscribing and restricting local beliefs and long standing practices similarly failed to address the felt needs of the people. These attempts by colonial governments which were supported in some cases by missionaries ran counter to the idea of religious freedoms articulated and championed by some western missionaries in Africa. Thirdly, we agree with Gray that these attempts in the past to proscribe traditional African religions exposed the state as being weak instead of the Gods which the states tried to eliminate. An indication of this reality is the long existence of the witches' villages to which many women have been confined as a result of local witch hunts which the state has not succeeded to eliminate. The embarrassment that these places still exist speaks to the failure of the attempts to police traditional remedies. We certainly do not endorse witch hunts in any way. But we recognize that in addressing the embarrassment of the reality of the witches' villages, most people have failed to recognize that the local priest in Gnani has been a stabilizing force for the many victims of witchcraft accusations. Several women emphasized in the interviews that they feel safe at Gnani because of the medicines they received from the priest. The work of the priest in the village is not only to conduct the divination to determine if the accused are guilty or not, but also to manage the affairs of the community and make sure that residents live peacefully. The services of the local priest had done a lot more to provide these women with peace of mind and calling him fetish priest actually engages in discrimination and a diabolization of the many services he has rendered to the residents of the village. The growing references to fetish practices to local priests like the one in Gnani amounts to what Fabien Eboussi Boulaga described as the missionary discourse which employs the language of derision and refutation (Boulaga 1981).

The history of Islam in the region, especially among the Dagomba, dates back to the 1800s. Contact was made with what was described during colonial times as Turkish religion, a reference probably to Islam, and in the 1820s some traders from Yendi are known to have indicated that the area was mostly Muslim or were governed by Koranic laws and the reality was recognized by both converts to Islam and non-converts (Wilks 1965). Scholars claim the Muhammad Zangina described as the first king of the Dagomba, even though other historical records claim he was the 16th ruler of the Dagomba, promoted Islam and Arabic leaning in his realm (Wilks 1965). Although Islam is described as Turkish religion, it is noted that the Hausas were in the area as there was a well-known trading route that brought them to the region and Zangina himself encouraged Hausa traders, malams, and artisans to settle in his realm and many of them settled in Kamshagu, which is not too far away from Yendi.

Other religious groups have started work in the area with the Methodists opening a church not too far away from the witches' village. At the location, in 2009 a Methodist Church of Ghana school was built by World Mission Possible. When we visited the village in June, we were told that there is a Catholic Church and a Baptist Church. The pastor of the Baptist Church served as interpreter for some of the interviews and both he and a lay leader in the Catholic Church served as assistants to the medical team that visited from World Mission Possible in 2015. As a sign of religious pluralism, we noted that the Baptist pastor is the brother of the local priest who receives people accused of witchcraft into the village. One could say that there are many more choices for the residents of the village when it comes to religion. This was evident to us because even if we did not ask them about their religion, some of the women were eager to tell us that there were Muslims or Christians. Several of the residents in the village have experienced a religious conversion during their stay in the village. For example, Elizabeth became a Christian in the camp and now attends the Baptist church. Some were already Muslims when they came and have remained practicing Muslims.

Religious leaders in Ghana today condemn the treatment of so-called witches who have been sent to live in witches' villages. In a study prepared by the Southern Sector of Youth and Women's Empowerment Network (SO-SYWEN), several religious leaders condemned the treatment of witches in Ghana. Shiekh Nuhu Shaributu, the National Chief Imam called for peaceful co-existence and respect for the elderly which is often ignored in witchcraft accusations. He called for authorities to work and educate the public on respect for other people, the law, and report abuse of people to the police. Togbe Adjah Kofi V, and Chief Tafi Mador of the Volta Region called on the Ghanaian Government to stop these outmoded practices through education and enforcement of the law. The Most Reverend Vincent Sowah Boi-Nai the Catholic Bishop of Yendi called on the state to work to stop these dehumanizing practices. The Reverend Dr. Fred Deegbe, the General Secretary of the Christian Council of Ghana argues that "women are virtuous and have many qualities that are beneficial to society as a whole. Like the trokosi system, let us all work towards abolishing any cultural practice that dehumanizes women and other vulnerable groups in our society." The trokosi system, which was abolished, was a practice where young women were given as brides to certain deities; a practice some have dated to the early 16th century. It was controversial because many saw it as ritual and sexual servitude and worked to abolish it in most of the places where the ritual was practiced. While there is no indication that the women who have been sent to the Gnani witches' village have been subjected to sexual abuse, the comparison here relates to the loss of freedom and confinement within a certain geographical space mainly on grounds that someone suspects that you are a witch.

While the spiritual fever of Pentecostalism might not have gripped Gnani with the force with which has taken the rest of the Ghanaian community, we noted that it is coming to the area. The new Methodist church which has opened in the area is very dynamic and the worship was very animated. The language and Pentecostal discourse is clearly present in this church and the lively music is an indication that many embrace the power of the Holy Spirit as proclaimed by the Pentecostals. But it would not surprise us if down the road a group of people could emerge in the church who offer services to exorcise people from the power of witchcraft as it is happening in other Ghanaian and Nigerian cities and contemporary studies of Pentecostalism in Ghana demonstrate that this might be the case in the near future. Pentecostal churches exist in the Yendi district and while we have not established specific responses to witchcraft from the Pentecostal tradition in the region, there are reasons for us to speculate that their teachings in the near future could affect the way people in the region think and respond to witchcraft. The teaching of the Pentecostal Churches on witchcraft has received academic discussion in the work of Pastor Opoku Onyinah, in *Pentecostal Exorcism: Witchcraft and Demonology in Ghana*, in which he discusses the staying power of belief in witchcraft.

The other way of understanding witchcraft discourses in Ghana and contemporary Africa has been advanced by Pentecostal church leaders. Some of their approaches attack everything they do not agree with, including other religious practices, merely on grounds that these are not Christian practices. Ghanaian Pentecostal pastor and academic Opoku Onyinah has attacked occultism in which he includes divination, spiritism, sorcery and magic, witchcraft and astral projection, witch demonology, *mami wata*, the occult youth, the occult crime, and occultism in government. Prior to discussing occultism in which he addresses witchcraft, he mischaracterizes, in our view, Post-Modernism as a false world view because postmodernist say that one cannot say if something is true or right. This does not reflect the debates on Post-Modernism and ignores the fact that many scholars of Post-Modernism are religious people who merely argue that the certainty of foundations constructed on the scaffolding of modernity may not hold as once believed. What Onyinah forgets is that the postmodern critique of modernity in a way re-inscribes religion for a different historical epoch. While no one in our team supports beliefs in witchcraft, lumping all those beliefs into demon possession has led to excesses in the Christian community where pastors and religious leaders have themselves engaged in abusive behavior in the name of exorcism.

If one were to ask Africans and non-Africans why Pentecostal churches and their proclamation of Pentecostal power is so captivated by witchcraft and the fact that many Africans still turn to traditional religious belief and practices; one would get different answers ranging from the persistence of so called outmoded beliefs and social norms. But we think Birgit Meyer offers a reasonable explanation for the ambivalent yet cantankerous relationship between Christianity and especially Pentecostalism to traditional beliefs and witchcraft. In "Translating the Devil," Meyer argues that missionaries treated local Ewe Gods as servants of the devil. In other words, missionaries recognized traditional deities (and one might add, the rituals carried out by priests who serve those deities) but it is just that those Gods serve the devil that has been constructed in Christianity and other religions. This "Pentecostalization" of the problem has led to different ministries of deliverance and exorcism, with the most recent being deliverance from witches by Pentecostal pastors in and out of Africa.

Other Pentecostal scholars argue that we should be careful today of relating everything, and in our case, African beliefs to demonology. Walter J. Hollenweger has argued that questions that surround demonology are difficult to resolve and one must be cautious in making any pronouncements on them (2005). Most of the religious leaders who do this equate the African world with the world view of the time when the bible was written, or treat views on spirits as if there were the same all over the world. Keith Warrington calls for more caution in equating everything one encounters in a non-Christian culture as part of demonology. Our perspective is that seeing everything about witchcraft through the lens of the New Testament and then arguing that all things that are not Christian must be of the devil has led some Christian leaders to see the remedies to witchcraft that are offered in places like Gnani as merely fetish practices. Accordingly, the local priest who administers the oracle and gives the women of have been accused of being witches is a fetish priest. We think that this kind of language does not encourage dialogue on the very crucial issues the women in the village face.

Listening to many of the women in Gnani reminded us of the key role the priest plays in their stabilization. Many of them said that although they were accused and rejected by their own relatives, when they came to Gnani, the priest declared them innocent. Those who did not use that language, which others might interpret as a tacit confession of guilt, said that the priest gave them medicines to defuse any negative powers. It is telling that when accused, either in colonial times, or in the postcolonial state, many of the women did not run to the state, or to the other religious communities who are now condemning the local priest. If we have any concerns here about the medicines the women say they have been given to detect witchcraft or treat a person so that he or she does not have any witchcraft again, our concerns stem largely from biomedical concerns. We wonder about the nature of the medicines the women are given to drink when they arrive at the village. Our curiosities here concern the chemical or therapeutic compounds of these medicines, which everyone in the NGO community and many government leaders refer to derisively as "concoction." As far as we can tell from our interviews, no one in the Gnani village has died from taking these medicines. If anything, they report that it has made them whole again. Although in 2004, in the Edo State of Nigeria, 27 men and women suspected of witchcraft died after being forced to drink some of these 'witch-finding concoctions' (Damasane 2009).

Residents take religious life seriously as we gathered from their remarks about religion. When we asked Merina if she believes in witchcraft, she not only said she did not believe in it, but told us that she prays to God and cannot kill anybody. She had been at the village for only 4 years. She was 40 years old at the time and was accused of using witchcraft to kill. At first when we asked if she did anything to the person she was accused of killing she just opened her hands and held them wide open and gestured in a way that said I am also surprised. She did not have a clue why she was accused and 4 years later, she still demonstrated the surprise that she was singled out for doing something she did not do. As far as she was concerned, being a Christian meant that one cannot kill another person, therefore she could not practice witchcraft. She told us that women do not have the power to counter these accusations and they are forced into these situations when they are not guilty. The woman we interviewed after her immediately associated witchcraft to the ability to kill someone. She told us, "I do not know how to kill someone." It is clear that she was still baffled by the accusation that she had killed someone.

Chapter Two

Gnani—Banished to Witches' Village

During the last two decades, the Ghanaian government, human rights activists, faith-led and non-governmental organizations (NGOs), and the international community have responded with shock to the reality that several villages in northern Ghana are designated "witches' villages." Many global entities, including the UNHCR, have expressed disapproval and outrage that these villages continue to exist in the twenty-first century.

In this chapter we will discuss in expansive terms what day-to-day life is like in one of the witches' villages, based on our six years of work in Ghana, and our five years of work and research within the village of N'gani in the Yendi municipality in northern Ghana. Much of the literature that examines the sites where individuals are accused of practicing witchcraft in northern Ghana have been referred to as "camps." In interviews given to scholars and non-governmental organizations (NGOs), some Ghanaian officials refer to settlements as "camps." We have chosen to use the term "village." The decision to use the term "village" does not contest any of the ideas associated with the term "camp" (such as a place where one is confined, or sent to live temporarily, or where a person experiences a certain loss of freedom which many of the residents have indeed experienced). We use the term "village" to maintain the dialectic of temporality and permanence which we think reflects the way many of the residents have come to view their lives in the village. Such a dialectical view allows us to see both the sense of temporality expressed in the acute sense of the loss of their homes (which the residents have expressed to us), and the equally strong view expressed by many of them that they want to remain in there until they die. In Gnani witches' village, the oppressed residents have cultivated a familiar shelter and refuge from trials, a space where they have conceded to a local truce—an imposed armistice if you will—in order to negotiate a peace and pacify their community.

In replacing the term "camp" with the term "village," we do not want to diminish or mitigate what clearly is a brutal subject matter—exile. They are in an encampment set aside for witches, but they also feel "safe" in a way that is inexplicable to visitors, but becomes clear when one gets to know these residents. We also prefer the term "village" because regardless of the intentions of the members of the various communities we believe what may have been designed as a temporary site (with harsh and stigmatizing conditions), has in fact evolved into a semi-structured community where many women, some men, and a growing number of children live their lives (on society's margins), adjusting to their new reality. The contestations which have arisen among contemporary Ghanaians are that many practices in these villages are "part of an old world" that they would prefer to forget. Finally, by calling them "villages" we do not seek to impose permanent status to these (temporary) resettlements, and along with the Ghanaian government and many other human-rights activists, we would also embrace a future that will cease to necessitate witches' villages.

This study therefore is a limited analysis of aspects of witchcraft in northern Ghana and focuses on the witches' village of Gnani. Mensah Adinkrah has argued that there is a larger world of witchcraft belief and alleged practice in Ghana and other places in Africa (2015). Adinkrah maps out the contemporary landscape of witchcraft in Ghana, which we found very informative. We do not consider that our focus on a singular witches' village skews our discussion, but merely comprehensively discusses aspects of the witchcraft in northern Ghana that dates back to the Colonial times and remains an existential dilemma as new so-called "witches" are admitted to these villages as you read this book. In doing so, we hope also that those who are engaged in dialogue about the witches' villages recognize that many places in Ghana and Africa share something in common: A symbolic approach to witchcraft that draws from spiritual powers. The only difference is that for some people today, addressing witchcraft is now within the spiritual domain of Christian leaders, who themselves use religious symbols and resources to manage it. Yet in Gnani, the predominant symbolic approach to witchcraft remains the work of the local priest. As authors, our goal is not to sensationalize this particular village, rather to revisit one locality and explore in dialogue with the residents of the witches' village their lives and the beliefs that led to their resettlement in the village. In so doing, we also explore the role of medicine, disease, illness, and healing as it has become clear to us that one cannot understand a social and spiritual phenomenon like witchcraft in isolation. Our appreciation for Adinkrah's recent study is the manner in which he has developed the theme of witchcraft violence, something communicated to us in the narratives provided by the residents of Gnani witches' village. Our study holds the idea of violence in a dialectical tension because the women are victims of violence which evicts, isolates, and banishes them from their homes into a life of exiled hardship. Yet as it will become clear, what was supposed to be a witches' wilderness has become a "home" of sorts for the impoverished women. Ironically, these are "homes" constructed in violence—yet the living conditions themselves reveal nothing to contemporary Ghanaians but a 'site of violence' rife in its marginalization and subsistence-level livelihood.

The witches' village in Gnani lies in the Yendi municipality in the Northern Region of Ghana. For an in-depth history of the region, authors Tamakloe (1931) and Oppong (1973) and Mahama (n.d.) have published books citing northern Ghana. The precise location of Gnani is approximately 14 miles to the north of Yendi. The village is covered with Savanah brushes and trees, foliage that is prevalent in the parched and arid region. The majority of the Gnani residents are farmers growing maize and yams, and/or raising goats for meat. The present chief of Gnani is Salifu Ziblim. He was preceded by Mahama Zakari who became chief in 1998 and died from a long-term illness on April 14, 2013. On April 14, 2013, my father passed on after a long-term illness. The Yendi municipality has a paramount chief whose palace is in the town of Yendi, a growing municipality that is also a promising center of commerce for the region. Scholars have proposed different dates for the founding and establishment of Yendi, but Shinnie and Ozanne argue that based on the chronology of the rulers, it is more likely that the town was settled in 1650 (1962). As in many parts of Ghana (and Africa) there are two systems of governance: the traditional which is headed by a chief (in the case of Yendi, a Paramount Chief); and the District Assembly, made up of elected representatives from the villages in the district. Today the Yendi municipality is represented in the Ghanaian Parliament by the Honorable Alhaji Mohammed Habibu Tijani, who served previously as the Chief Executive for the Yendi municipality for eight years.

The region has gone through years of violence with the most recent being the inter-ethnic violence that took place from 1980 through 1999 (Brukum 2001). Brukum has further argued that one of the violent episodes was sparked by a disagreement over something as insignificant as a disagreement over the price of a mango, which quickly escalated when a woman was killed. This incident immediately reawakened offended feelings on past disagreements, and precipitated violence between the Konkomba and Bimoba people. After local tensions had somewhat diminished, in March of 2002, the Ya Na, King of Dagbon, was murdered along with 30 other people. His body was then burned and dismembered, and then parts of his corpse were brandished around the city by his enemies who publicly rejoiced at the killings (MacGaffey 2006; Akudugu and Mahama 2011). Although these conflicts correlate to longstanding rivalries, unsubstantiated rumors began to be spread that the Dagbon caused these tensions in order to gain economic advantages (Agyekum 2002). These conflicts reflect a history of power disputes that have taken place in the region since Colonial times, and intensified in the 1930s when the Colonial government attempted to impose a remedy. Some observers of the region believe that the crises of the previous decades were a marked continuation of these regional tensions. However, some have argued that recent acts of violence in the region could be attributed to Post-Colonial Ghanaian national political disputes and struggles, but even here, most think the political contests reflect differences between the two ethnic groups and their long struggle for dominance or spirit of independence from each other. Regardless of what position one takes, the violence in 2002 embarrassed the government, especially then Vice President, Aliu Mahama, who was from Yendi where he had served in the District Council and an Assemblyman. It is estimated that the Ghanaian Government spent a total of six billion Ghanaian cedis to keep peace in the region after the violence (Brukum 2001). The Ghanaian government and international NGOs have promoted conflict resolution in the area and the Yendi Municipality is thriving again and businesses are growing in the region and a major road construction that will facilitate travel between Yendi and Accra, by-passing Tamale, is under construction.

According to 30-year-old Alidu Zakari, who is the son of the late chief of Gnani, his royal 25-member Ghanaian family has a powerful, deep-rooted history in this remote region of Ghana. Zakari explained the village's history as the following:

> In the 17th century, history had it that it was a place where mysterious trees and stone were gathered without the intervention of humans. On one occasion, a hunter walked a distance from Gnani to where these trees and stone are, to hunt for bush meat. When the hunter got there, he saw that the place was amazing since those trees and stones were gathered without human intervention. Also he found the tail of a cow and a calabash full of water and some herbs and bark of some specific trees. The hunter did not hunt, but carried the items to the chief. After showing it to the chief, it was decided that it was something that could be used to protect the community against spiritual problems. The reason behind this was that trees and stones are known as psychic protectors. The chief then created a strong psychic to implement this as a customary wall built between the village and the 'spiritual forest' of the village. In a trial, the hunter drank from calabash and began to speak unfamiliar things that were supposed to happen in the village to the people. He then became the information carrier from the "spirit world" to the people. When this behavior of the hunter continued for some couple of months, they came into agreement that the hunter should go and settle near the sacred forest where the calabash was found and there he was crowned as the "*Tindana*" which means "witch doctor" so the name of the village was called "*Gnani-Tindang*" or the witches' village. (Zakari interview 2008)

Since 2008 Zakari has worked with World Missions Possible as a translator and medical technician. The organization provided Zakari with medical training at Ankaase Faith Healing Hospital, medical books and some medical equipment, enabling Zakari to periodically check on Gnani resident's minor medical needs. Over eight years, we were able to conduct two separate research interviews with some of the residents of the Gnani witches' village. The first set of interviews were conducted by Zakari. The interviews were conducted in Gnani village in the two local languages spoken by residents of the witch's village, Dagbani, spoken by the Dagbani people and Likpakpaln, Kpankpan, and Kom Komba, the language of the Konkomba. Both interviews were conducted in light of the IRB approved by Rice University research division which specified that women residents in Gnani witches' village would be interviewed. For these interviews, we sought the permission of the past and current chief of Gnani and they gave their approval. The forms were subsequently read to Shei Alhassan, the *Tindana,* (priest) who is in charge of the witch's village, and he gave us his permission. The interviews were then explained to the women who volunteered to be interviewed and they signed the forms. These were semi structured interviews and during the longer interviews, Bongmba asked them questions which invited the women to tell their stories and also responded to specific questions. Bongmba's questions were translated into the local language spoken by the respondent. The translators for these interviews were Zakari and Shei Fushein, the Baptist Pastor in the village, who is the younger brother of the *Tindana.* He is a skilled gentleman who did not have many years of formal education, but recruited and trained as a pastor in a Bible School in Uganda. Zakari has served as both a translator and a medical technician trainee for World Mission Possible and other NGOs for many years.

During our visit to the village in 2015, Bongmba and Zakari, the research assistant, visited the chief. The little village is ruled under the leadership of a chief referred to as "*Gnani-dana,*" meaning the chief of Gnani. We arrived in the hall where the chief receives visitors and guests first. We sat down and were greeted by four nobles from the village. Shortly after that the chief arrived and we all stood up and greeted him. He was very well dressed for the occasion. He welcomed us to the village and Zakari introduced Bongmba and told him that Bongmba was friends of Dr. Thomas Flowers and Dr. Roxane Richter of World Mission Possible and that he had come to the area to do research on the witches' village. It was during this visit that he gave us his permission and advised us to first visit the *Tindana,* and get his permission as well. He was very delighted to know that the medical team would be coming to his village again.

The witches' village lies on the outskirts of the main town of Gnani and slopes down gently to the plains. The small mud-baked houses (or huts) are grouped in small clusters. The house of the *Tindana* is located at the end of the settlement near the ritual complex that also has a shrine where divination takes place. The *Tindana* is the one who accepts new residents into the village; therefore he is the head of the witches' village, but the Chief of the town of Gnani has legal jurisdiction over the entire area. The *Tindana*, as priest, is the ritual leader of the witches' village. In that capacity, he plays an important role in the lives of the residents and is the person they all turn to if something goes wrong. He is the intermediary between the residents of the witches' village, and the rest of Gnani village. He has been called different names by visitors and religious leaders from different religious traditions. For example some call him, "witchdoctor" a colonial expression that does not really tell us very much about the office he occupies. Christian pastors, some who joined the medical team two days later call him "fetish priest." The current *Tindana* is a middle-aged man, probably in his early 50s. He is married and lives in the village with his wife and children.

When Bongmba initially arrived, there were a group of students visiting from one of the local schools in the region. The students and their teacher were being given a briefing on the village by the resident priest. The attention the witches' villages have received means that people visit these villages regularly. Their deliberations continued for about an hour and when they left, Zakari introduced Bongmba to the *Tindana*, and he greeted us warmly and welcomed us to the village. All the other people, mostly men who were gathered in the court yard greeted us and carried on a conversation with Zakari in the local language. The *Tindana* was pleasantly surprised when he was told that Bongmba was born and grew up in Cameroon. Bongmba felt that the excitement in the crowd spoke more to the kinship that he shared with them especially on the question of witchcraft since he has studied witchcraft among his own people, the Wimbum people of the Northwest Province of Cameroon. The *Tindana* gave his consent and called the senior resident and talked with her and she said that she would sign the consent form for the other residents who would be willing to talk with Bongmba.

But Bongmba also noted that he thought he had a good knowledge of the village from previous accounts from Flowers, Richter, and Zakari, and also read previous interviews and documents related to the research and work of World Mission Possible, but he was not prepared for the surprise. The sprawling and sloping village was larger than Bongmba expected. He was taken aback by seeing so many children growing up in a supposed witches' village, especially given the stigma attached to it. Additionally, there were far more women than he expected. Bongmba says that he did not know what to expect, even after talking with many women who have been accused of practicing witchcraft in Cameroon. But there he was in a world which he thought could not be any further from human imagination, yet the community was an imagined community if one were to invoke Benedict Anderson's well-received idea, it was an imagined community, but one that was conceptualized and structured on an exclusive agenda which targeted some members of a former community on suspicion that they were witches, and then proceeded to exclude them and they in turn found a new community, reserved for so-called witches (Anderson 2006).

One of the women from the compound served us local beer. The beer tasted wonderful, and Bongmba found out that it was made in the village and he offered to buy some and share with the people gathered in the courtyard that morning. He asked Zakari to inquire if this would be acceptable since he did not want to drink alone. The priest simply joked that if Bongmba spent a million cedis, they could not refuse to drink it. At this first meeting, the *Tindana* explained what takes place in very basic terms to dispel wrong information about what happens at the village. He emphasized that contrary to what some people think, they do nothing to recruit people to the village. They merely provide a safe place for those who have been accused of practicing witchcraft, who have been rejected, and threatened with violence, to stay in peace. He said that all the women who have come to the village are searching for peace and here they find a place where they can sleep and not worry that something will happen to them. Speaking through the translators, he said: "My desire is that regardless of what has been said about them, when they come here, they will leave all of those things behind them and live here in peace." He further said that when the women arrive, he conducts divination to determine if they are witches. Many times he does not even bother to find out, because the medicines he gives them are very strong and help neutralize the witchcraft in them. He stated that this ritual process was responsible for the peace and calm that prevails in the community.

Our contacts and direct conversations with the residents of Gnani witches' village go back several years. Since 2008, we have gathered information that presents a complex demographic profile. The majority of the people in the Gnani village are women and we have talked with many of the residents but carried out one-on-one interviews with 95 residents in various sessions. The initial detail interviews were done with 63 women and 1 man in 2008, with follow-up discussions during subsequent visits. In 2015, we conducted an additional 31 semi-structured interviews again with several women of the village in either their residence, or the premises of the group's spokesperson. Some of the interviews were conducted during the days the medical clinic was held—as a convenience for interviewees who insisted they did not want to lose their coveted place in line. Even in that context, we did everything to respect the privacy of the participants. Two could only talk during the break at the clinic and the only place where we could ensure their privacy was to hold the meeting in one of our two vans. These were long semi-structured interviews in which we asked two types of questions. The first type of question gave the residents an opportunity to give factual information such as the number of years the person had lived in the village, and information about family, religion, and things which we found out were very important to the villagers. Despite the fact that they had been forced from their homes, nearly all of the women spoke about their families, making several references to their husbands, children, grandchildren, co-wives, step children, in-laws, fathers, mothers, and other relatives. One would have thought that stigma might have erased these more intimate and familial terms, but the terms remained and the residents of Gnani referred to people by these relationships. The second form of questions were open-ended queries. For example, they were asked to describe what happened before they came to Gnani. This often gave them the freedom to give an account and in the ensuing dialogue they expressed themselves, sometimes with great humor, and at other times with solemnity and/or visible anger. All the women interviewed in 2015 indicated that they were 'exonerated' by the local priest as the divination performed cleared them from the accusations.

MAPPING A COMMUNITY CONSTRUCTED ON STIGMA

During our interviews we came up with a general profile of some of the residents of the village. For example, from the group we interviewed, Binetu, the longest resident, had spent 35 years at Gnani village, and Mairo had been living in the village for only 3 months. (Note: all names of our research interviewees are fictitious.) The fact that someone had been there for only three months was a grim reminder to us that while the debate rages about what to do about the witches' village, new residents who have been accused continue to arrive. Therefore, despite the national and international attention the villages have received, they continue to admit new residents who have been accused of practicing witchcraft. For instance, in 2015, we arrived shortly after a new resident had been admitted, and we were able to witness a group of women escorting her to her new dwelling.

Therefore the average number of years (in all interview sessions and years) of the condemned Gnani "witches" and one "warlock" was 14.7 years; thus an average between 16.6 years (in the 2008 interview session) and 10.9 years (in 2015 interviews). Consequently, we should underscore the idea that despite what government officials' claim—Gnani witches' village is currently an active and growing community.

Most of the women we interviewed came from different villages within the (northern) Yendi municipality. The translators estimated that the woman who had traveled the longest distance to come to Gnani came from Wulensi, a town in Nanumba south district, about 60 miles away from Gnani village. The resident from the closest village had traveled only 10 miles to come to Gnani. Although they all talked about family in our 2015 interview session, only 13 women out of our 31 sample group told us the number of children they had; they had given birth to 68 children and 11 of them were no longer alive. Miriam, who had lived in the village for 20 years, gave birth to a child at the Gnani village. Exile to Gnani was a punishment and an act that isolated the residents from the rest of their families. We were given the impression that most of the women do not see their relatives or maintain any contacts with them. Eleven of the women reported that their relatives do visit them. The visitors included a brother of one of the residents, one grandson, and the rest of the visitors were the children of the residents, and one of them reported that her children live with her at the Gnani village, although we do not know if this was a permanent living arrangement. For the most part, the women whose husbands were still alive reported no contact with them and no conjugal visits.

According to Zakari, a son of the former (now deceased) Gnani chief, the women have a leader to represent them and she is usually a woman who has spent several years at a village, and such is the case in Gnani. He stated:

> The witches' village has a leader called *Magaziya*, who represents them. She is the 'voice of the witches' and it is her responsibility is to carry information from the witches to the chiefs and the witchdoctor whenever they encounter a problem in the village. Witches and wizards are not allowed to roam freely outside the camp. This explains the reason why the witchdoctor has his hut where the concoctions are kept [nearby] in the vicinity. The shrine is built with a special hut where in a small round room where all the jujus and the concoctions are kept for the [trials] proves and tests of the alleged witches and wizards. However, no one goes in there and no one touches it except the witchdoctor and his family members. (2015)

She became a spokesperson for the group out of necessity because there was no one to lead and speak on behalf of the women or organize the community and keep peace. She volunteered and continues to serve as leader. She does not remember exactly what year she came to the village as a victim of witchcraft accusation, but thinks that at the time she arrived, the present *Tindana* might have been a youth, perhaps a teenager. She has seen most of the residents of the village arrive in the village, go through the intake, settle, and become active members of the community. She therefore has seen the community grow. Given the attention witches' villages have received in Ghana and internationally, they have been speaking openly about their experience, circumstances, and demanding that local politicians and the Ghanaian government do something about their plight in the village. When non-governmental organizations come the leader is the one who speaks on behalf of the women. The women who come to the village can go back, but many of the women who have settled in Gnani witches' village do not plan to leave the village. Some of the younger women live with their husbands and have children in the village.

The following are excerpts from our one-on-one interview sessions with Gnani condemned "witches" residents beginning in 2008:

- They call me here Mima Fati. In fact, I have been in this camp for 14 year long. Before I was brought here, I was very strong enough to do certain things on my own. But when I came here I lose strength simply because I do not get enough food to eat, not to talk of having enough rest. So, I hope you [World Missions Possible] would continue to take good care of us to survive in the remaining years we are to spend in this world. Thank you.
- My name is Klumbei. I am seventy (70) years old. My granddaughter died for about four (4) years ago and my own children said I was the one who was responsible for her death. For that, they said they can't live with me anymore. So I was brought here to stay and suffer as they supposed of me. However, I really suffered different ways. But now when World Missions Possible came and offered drugs and medical treatment, I see changes in my life. So I would like to thank them for the help assistance they gave me. Thank you.
- I, Rahaman, want to express sincere gratitude and thanks to the World Mission Possible for the first but continues help they have promised going me in the witches' camp. However, I have been here for about three (3) years ago, and there was not any assistance given to me, until they came with drugs and other medical equipment to see the health of we, the accused witches, at the witches camp in N'gani in the Yendi district. In fact, after they offered us the drugs, we have been in good health. We have seen great changes in our health and we regained a lot of strength in order to continue some of our farming activities. Furthermore, we have nothing doing here thank help people in their farming activities to enable us get some by day money to survive. So I thank the doctors concerned for the health assistance they gave us.
- My name is Adam. Though I am still a young but grown woman. But I was accused by my brother of killing his son. For that matter I was brought here to traditionally wash my stomach as they say (remove the witchcraft from me). But when I finish washing my stomach, they say I shouldn't come home. And now I am suffering very seriously, and I would be happy to have more of your help. As for as I have promised to be faithful to you. Bye!
- I am called Wumbei. I am in the witches' camp here in Gnani for six (6) years now. In fact, I have encountered health problem until when I got information from my colleagues that the World Mission Possible was coming to check on the health in the camp. I did not waste time, but rushed to the center and I was given some drugs to be taken. However since the time I took the drugs I have not experience any health problems up till now. I therefore pray and wish that the world mission possible would come back here and give us the necessary assistance, especially our health. Thank you.
- Mahama is my name. I am 63 years old. I have been here for about seven (7) years ago. My brother was seriously ill and his back-borns who were twins said I was responsible for the illness and so therefore I was forcefully sacked from our house to come here and drink the spiritual water they have in the shrine here. When we came they said I shouldn't follow them home. I remained here. Actually I have encountered enough problems as I am here. But I thank World Mission Possible for their kind support they gave me on

the part of my health for a couple months ago. I still hope that they would not stop helping us. Thank you.

- I am Iddisu. I am fifty (50) years old. I am here for about five years ago. I have nothing to say than to say that my families all told a lie on me for killing my brother's son. So they neglected me and brought me here forever. But I pray that you will continue to come here and give us the necessary help as you did ago. Greetings to Doctor Roxane and colleagues.
- I am called Pagwuni. I have stayed here for about four (4) years today. I have been praying seriously to get somebody who will help me in all means here. But now I hope that the World Missions Possible have opened their help to me. Foremostly, they gave me medical treatment when I first saw them in the camp. So I hope they will continue helping us. Thank you.
- My name Azindo. I am 48 years old. I have been here for three (3) years ago. I was brought here accidentally by the death of my family brother in which his brothers and sisters accused me of being the killer of him. When they brought me here, four years ago, they never mind coming to see how I live here. So I hope that you would take good care of me till I die here. Because I can't not go back to them. They will kill me if I go there.
- My name is Adam Pagnaa. I am 46 years old. I have been here for six (6) years ago. In fact, I don't have much to say about the experience I had here. I was wandering from herb to herb for my head but when the World Missions Possible came and the doctors, especially the doctor who was a lady, at my first sit took good look at me and patiently check and made a good prescription for me, I recovered very normal. So I pray that, it should not the last and first time they will visit us here. Thank you.
- My name is Yakubu. In fact I have been here through a suspect from people of been a witch so my own son brought me here traditionally in order to prevent further havoc to him and the family as a whole. But I wish I had gone back to him because I am suffering here.
- I am called Ziblim. I am 63 years old. I have been here for about one year ago. Actually I have find life not easy for that short stay in the camp. So I pray that World Mission Possible would come to my help in order not suffer more for I will stay for long time here.
- My name is Adam. I am 70 years old. In fact I know I am not too old to do few things on my own. But I am appealing to the doctors from World Missions Possible to still provide their help on me to enable me to be a healthy old lady. I pray that God will richly bless them and Alidu. Thank you.
- I am called Budali. I am thirty three (33) years old. I have been in the camp for about four (4) years ago. I don't have anything to say, but only to thank the World Missions Possible for sympathizing us here in the camp. I would like to say that without your help some of us would have died through illness and hunger. So I still wish you would continue to attend to us help here in the camp. Thank you.
- My name is Amadu. I have nothing to say then to thank the World Mission Possible for the kind of concern they have on us here. In fact we were here helpless, but now we are now in the mood of happiness since we first saw the World Mission Possible.

- Yakubu is my name. I am fifty three (53) years old. I was staying near Yendi a village called Kpatuya. However, my misfortune started when a young man from our village died through a sickness. However, the young man's father called my children and told them that they suspected me of been the killer of that young man. Traditionally when you are accused of being a witch, they normally send you to the shrine to prove yourself innocent of having witchcraft. So we did that and Gnani Shrine and I was finally accused that, was really having the witchcraft. Therefore they said that I shouldn't come back to the village. Hence I am here in the village for about eight (8) years now. Furthermore, my health was a big problem for me until the World Mission Possible came a couple of months ago and came to us aid on the health part. Therefore, I would like to express my sincere love to the World Missions Possible for the assistance they gave me.

- As for me, I was in my room when they came to burn my room. When I waked up and asked them why they wanted to set my room on fire, they replied that they suspected I was a witch. So therefore, I was forced to leave my village for Gnani to join the witches. However, when I first came here I was strong but now I am weak. So I appeal to many at World Missions Possible to come to my aid to help me regain the strength I was having. I also want to thank the doctors for the medical examination they took me through during the time they came to the centre here in Gnani. I say God bless you all and that of our own grandson Alidu. Thank you.

- My name is Napare. I am 51 years old. I am a woman who has been living with my uncle after I lost my husband. However, I was with him when one of his children who was a boy was seriously sick and was sent to a herbalist for local treatment. He was there for some number of months when there was not any changes with him, so they brought him back home and he died with the illness. Furthermore, after his death, my uncle called me and told me that I was the one who did magic and kill the boy, was really the person who killed the boy, he said he went and soothsayed from a soothsayer. Two days later, I was asked to leave the village. For the witches came at N'gani. In fact, I have stayed for about thirteen (13) years now in N'gani. And all my family has neglected me. I faced the following problems: 1) Health—when I am sick there is nobody to take care of me, 2) Food—I don't have enough supply of food, 3) Shelter—Where I live is very poor environment, don't even have better clothings to wear, not to talk of getting good water to drink.

- I am called Abdulai. I am sixty six (66) years old now. I have been here for about twenty (20) years now. Because of that, I missed my family for many years. However, I was very strong when I was brought here and one juju woman who claimed to be somebody who could detect somebody who has witchcraft powers. As of now I would like to say that I have benefited a lot from World Missions Possible. Thus the medical treatment I had from you has energize me a lot. I therefore thank you very well and may God strongly bless you.

- I am called Mariyama. But popularly they call me Mariyam. In fact, there is nothing I can say but only that of my brother who suspected me of been a witch and brought me here. I know it was a lie he told on me, but there was

not any escape to me than to accept what he say. I was brought here
accompanied with strong men with severe beatings till we reach here. So I
thank you very much for showing concern on us. Thank you.

While a majority of the residents are women who live alone, several members of the community have families that live with them, and some of the
children attend school. We asked the leader if the husbands came with their
wives when they were expelled from their respective villages. She said that it
is not the case that the husbands come with their wives, except in a few cases,
but some of the women meet other men when they have moved to the village
and marry them. When we expressed surprise, she smiled and wondered why
we talking as if we do not know that "you can find love anywhere" you look.

THE LOGIC OF A WITCHES' VILLAGE

The history of the witches' village is well known in Northern Ghana and
some claim that they have existed for over 100 years. The witches' village of
Kpatinga was started just about the time Ghana was gaining its indepen-
dence. Other villages include Kukuo village, which was the basis of the film
"Witches in Exile." Gambaga witches' village, which according to reports
houses over 700 female residents, is the subject of the documentary film
"The Witches of Gambaga." Other villages include Bonyase, Nabuli, and
Gnani (the focus of this study). Central to the recent discourses about condemned witches' villages is the question of human rights and freedoms.
Local and outside non-governmental organizations and academics have addressed the question of the witches' village and given the prevailing sentiments which not only condemn the existence of these villages, but call for
their immediate dismantlement.

One cannot argue that only women have been accused of being witches,
but it is the case that even from the beginning, women bore the brunt of most
the accusations. Firstly, women who were accused and condemned for allegedly being witches were sent to one of these villages as a punishment. From
this perspective, one could argue that for women, the witches' village func-
tioned like a penal colony where those who were accused were sent to serve
time. The women who have been sent to these villages have lost their freedom to live in their own homes and are made to live in a place they do not
consider home. Secondly, it seems to us, that some of the women who are
accused are sent to the witches' village as part of a political bargain with the
family or village. Since there is a perception in the area that witches are evil
persons who do things that can cause harm, harboring such a person in the
village would be considered collaborating with, supporting, or abating the
alleged evil acts they are accused of doing. Therefore family members do not
have very much leverage in providing support for the accused person. Thus if

a family member wanted to live in peace in the village, they have to send away the accused person to the witches' village. This scenario is precisely what happened in the case of Maimona. When her husband died, she moved back to live with her father. Unfortunately, her father died after some time while she was living in her father's compound. Maimona was later accused of killing her nephew, who had become ill and died. When we asked if her brother came to her defense, she said he did not, because he feared for his life and therefore asked Maimona to go to the witches' village and take the medicines that would prove her innocence. However, her brother did nothing further to support, augment, or ensure her safety and/or welfare. In contexts where the male members of the family exercise authority over the women, Maimona had no choice but to comply and go to the witches' village. Oftentimes, the claims of witchcraft against widowers can be directly associated to land disputes, domestic finances, and/or battles over inherited familial property. Thirdly, several women indicated that they escaped to the witches' village as they feared for their safety, and in their escape they found the witches' village to be a safe sanctuary for themselves (and others like them) who had been socially condemned by their communities.

Since the village was designed as a space where the witches would be isolated, it was not a surprise for us to hear several residents report that their relatives do not visit them. Those who reported that they have been visited or do have regular visits, or go back themselves to their former villages to visit were small. The leader and spokesperson for the residents of the village in Gnani told us that she sometimes pays a visit to her former home town. We have not established specific reasons why and how she is able to do this, but a number of things make this attitude understandable. She has lived at Gnani village for about 45 years, and is probably in her seventies. If our speculation about her age is correct, she has reached an age where she has authority as a mother and grandmother to assert herself, even in a patriarchal context. Her village is only 14 miles from Gnani. But we also suspect that since she has served as spokesperson for the rest of the villagers, she has also acquired the skill to speak for herself and take a stand on issues that she would not have taken several years ago. When we asked what it is like for her to go back to the village from which she was driven out, she said that most people do not like to see her and some do not even talk to her. Only her brother agrees that she should come to visit and assures her that nothing will happen to her. In other words, her social stigma of 'being a witch' has not been effectively extinguished.

Maimona also told us that although life in the village was peaceful, it was a challenge to find and provide food especially for her grandchildren who had come to live with her. We asked if they were not afraid of living with her in the witches' village, and she said that the children are not afraid. She pointed out that there are many other children living in Gnani. However, her grandchildren are young and unable to contribute towards the already insufficient food supply. So Maimona plants and grows modest patches of maize, yams, and vegetables in a marginal effort to nutritionally sustain herself and her growing grandchildren.

ACCUSED AND DECLARED GUILTY

Our account draws largely from the accusations that have been reported by the women themselves. This approach provides us a singular viewpoint from which we can analyze the complex world of the witches' village. We want to underscore that this represents one perspective on witchcraft discourses and beliefs on witchcraft, as we have not included the very significant dimension of witchcraft: Confessions that have been part of the analysis of witchcraft by Africanists in and outside Ghana (Debruner 1961; Fields 1960; Wyllie 1973; Field 1940; McLeod 1957; Douglas 1970; Dovlo 2007). R.E. Wyllie argued several years ago that the Effutu people believe in witchcraft but do not directly accuse others of bewitching them. Rather, they seek help from a priest *okomfo,* who will give them protective medicines (Wyllie 1973). Sometimes the medicines can also affect witches and cause them to self-accuse. This perspective reflects what happens in many contexts because in some communities, people do not make an accusation until they have consulted a diviner. When the diviner indicates that someone is the source of misfortune, the community then confronts the person and sometimes the person confesses. We do not know if any of current residents of Gnani confessed that they were witches. We do not have any data on such confessions. What we were told many times by the residents is that they did not do what they were accused of doing. From our conversations, we also know that the women did not confront their accusers and/or forcefully reject the accusations leveled against them. When we pressed them about the accusations, several only said they do not know anything about witchcraft.

When the accused is moved out of their home or village, very distinctive customs and specific members of a community are called upon in order to to "safely" transport the individual suspect. Zakari explained some parts of the process involved in the accused witch's transportation and trials (also referred to as "proves" by the indigenous people) in the Gnani village:

> In the case of Gnani, the chief will authorize his messenger called "*Naacham-lana*" to lead them to the witchdoctor. This is a person known to have the spiritual powers that render witches and wizards powerless. He lives near the shrine where sacrifices to the gods are done. The shrine is the place where the "proves" [trials] and sacrifices are done to confirm the reality of the witchcraft powers on anyone [who has] been accused. This sacrifice is done using chickens and other animals as instruments of the shrine. Incantations are believed to

be the spiritual language spoken and heard between the gods and the fetish priest in the shrine. This is done immediately after the oath. After the incantation, the chickens are killed. When a chicken falls on its back, it means that the person is successful and therefore possesses no witchcraft powers. But when the chicken falls on its belly, it indicates a positive accusation, and they bring some amount of money to be paid to the fetish priest for challenging the authority of the shrine and of the gods. (2015)

It is important to pay attention to cases that involve self-confessing witches, but this study discussed only the claims made by the women who consider themselves victims of false accusations. These accusations could have been related to the fact that something unusual happened and people thought that something must have caused it (Pool 1989). The accusations that forced them out of their homes varied. Three women were accused of killing their husbands and two were accused of killing their own sons. Two women were accused of killing their nephews and three were accused of killing other relatives (grandmother of her husband, another a stepson, and one was accused of killing a grandson). Five women were accused of killing their in-laws (brothers- or sisters-in-law). Eight women said that they were accused of killing "someone" and when we asked if they knew the person they were accused of killing, they only stated to us that they did not know. The last three types of accusations were positioned in a dissimilar category. Four women said that some people in their village saw the accused women in their dreams, and the villagers proceeded to accuse those women seen in dreams of being witches. Out of the four, two women reported that they were accused of causing two people to become ill. They were sent away, even though those people are still alive today.

Although we did not pursue the question of confession directly, that does not mean that we have concluded that people do not make such confessions in Gnani or other parts of the Northern Ghana. Instead, we decided to ask the women we interviewed if they believed that witchcraft exists. When asked that question, most of the residents of the village said they did not know. The closest answer to a belief that witchcraft exists was given by a resident who merely claimed that she liked staying at Gnani because the medicines administered by the *Tindana* have the power to cleanse a person. When we pressed the question if she herself has witchcraft, she then categorically stated that she did not believe that anything exists like witchcraft. When we followed up that question and asked why people believe it and she told us "I cannot say because it is individual beliefs. People know why they believe it exists." We must also emphasize that our study was initiated in the context of medical outreach and our aim was neither to establish a historical connection to the illnesses or witchcraft, nor to address the question of guilt and confession, but rather to study the circumstances and/or reasons that the women were brought to the village, and learn more to about their experiences. Given the fact that some of the women of Gnani had lived and died in the village, we assume that some of them in the past would have gone to the village before the independence of Ghana, whereas at the time the rituals of witch-cleansing was fashionable in Northern Ghana.

Elsewhere Tachira, a condemned "witch" living in the Gambaga camp lost count of the number of rituals she went through during her 14-year-long "cleansing period" (Npong 2014). She was forced to pay for many of her rituals and trials, tasks that drained her of the last cedis of her widower savings. The only option left to her, Tachira said, was to finally acquiesce to the witchcraft allegations and to walk 59 miles to the Gambaga camp for safety:

> None of my denials would make them change their perception of me. I was eventually obligated to go through rituals meant to test my innocence. In the process, I was stripped naked, shaved, and walked through the market center for three days. Then I was confined. The majority of these rituals were performed at night. I was subjected to beating, molestation, and threats. Bitter concoctions were forced down my throat, and in some instances I was starved, in hopes that I would admit to being responsible for what I was being accused of. (Npong 2104, 2)

Npong points out that oddly enough, even though she's been 'cleared' of witchcraft, Tachira voluntarily remains in the Gambaga camp instead of attempting to reintegrate into her Ghanaian home village where they tortured and abused her over 14 years, saying: "What I passed through, it was more than hell" (Npong 2014, 4).

Hence, the majority of the Gnani residents refuse to even consider returning to their respective homes, planning to die in Gnani. Zakari explains the complex tradition of practices and rituals conducted when a condemned witch dies while residing in Gnani:

> Traditionally when a witch or a wizard dies, the witchdoctor would have to inform the chief of the village so that arrangements would be made for the burial of the person. Before this can be done, a member of the family of the deceased would be invited to witness the burial—but he or she does not take part in the process. However, a burial service is done in two categories which depending upon the condition under which the witch died. So if a witch dies during the time they would have been drinking the [trial or proving] concoction, it is believed that he or she has challenged the gods and died badly. In such situations the burial is done by tying a robe on the legs of the deceased and pulling him or her into the grave dug for the burial. When this happens they will be singing some traditional songs that praise the shrine. At this burial, family members of the deceased are not invited to witness the burial services. If a witch or wizard dies badly, no recommended traditional or religious funerals are performed for him or her. (2015)

The pattern of accusations against the women who were expelled from their homes and sent to Gnani focused on illness and death. This is the one thing that comes up in studies of witchcraft in other parts of Ghana and most of Africa. Witches are believed to do many things, but the one thing people fear most is the notion that witches allegedly have the power to cause illness and also cause the death of someone. The pattern of accusation was also consistent with what we know of studies of witchcraft since many people tend to hold the view that a witch can only hurt his or her relative, or people with whom they share residence, or live in the same village. In other parts of Africa if a witch wants to hurt a non-relative, he or she has to establish a link with that person either by giving these people those materials acquired through witchcraft powers, or lure them to share the spoils, or eat the human flesh that witches reportedly eat (Bongmba 2001).

Some of the accusations involved co-wives. In one case a co-wife accused Martha of trying to kill her. The co-wives' accusation was based on dreams she had. Martha denied the charge but her son advised her to leave and helped in bringing her to the witches' village. When she asked her son why he was doing this, he simply said that he could not stay with her in the village any longer. It is not clear if by that statement he too had concluded that his mother was guilty of the accusation. But he indicated that he thought his mother did not want to make peace with the accusers. This is a complex story for two reasons. First, the accuser did not suffer any injury. She only complained that she saw Martha, her co-wife, in her dreams and she suspected that Martha was trying to kill her. Second, one wonders if this was a case of jealousy on the part of the accuser. In either case, the accused also pointed out that their husband was no longer alive.

In our second case that involved co-wives, the co-wife of Rekia accused her of killing her son. She left the house to go fetch water and when she returned, she saw a crowd beating their husband. They had accused Rekia in her absence and apparently the husband did not agree. She decided to come to the witches' village to be purified. We were curious to know what she thought of witchcraft since she said she had come to be purified. At that point there was a conversation in the local language between the translators. Two other women approached the area where we were conducting the interview and did not wait for their turn, but just joined us, and furthermore, offered their opinion. They said that they thought that Rekia was subjected to injustice that cannot be pushed away by simply thinking that this was a matter of jealousy between co-wives. When we asked her if she was a witch, Rekia spoke through the interpreter and said: "I do not have it. I do not know if others have it." When we asked about state intervention in these cases, the women spoke among themselves again and told us that we should forget about it because the government is not going to do anything about witchcraft accusations. We pointed out that we hear the Ghanaian government is beginning to close some of the camps. We further probed them about making their voices known to state officials and she said, maybe if they write letters something can be done about their plight.

In another one of the accounts about dreams, Regina said that a boy had said that he had a dream and saw Regina in his dream. However, the boy did not show any symptoms of illness; he had merely shared his dream with other community members. The next day, Regina was asked to leave. Her grandson spoke on her behalf, but members of the community ordered him to take her to the witches' village. Her husband had died several years before this. She said that he was a 'tough' man and a member of the royal family. She said that if her husband were alive he would not have supported this action against her. Even the chief of the village did not do anything. When asked why the chief did not intervene, she told us that the chief simply said that he wanted her to be safe. The chief also thought it would be good for her to go away and drink the medicines that would be given to her at the witches' village. If her departure was framed as a precautionary action, we asked if the chief or any of the elders from the village had come to visit her and make arrangements for her to return to the village since nothing ever happened to the child who saw her in her dreams. She told us no one has come to see her. She also told us that her nephew lives in the village because her sister's husband was accused of witchcraft and he came to live in the village.

Some of the residents themselves narrated their stories in a manner that demonstrated that they knew that the villagers who accused them had all the information wrong. Rosemary told us that she believed that witchcraft exists, but insisted that she does not have it. We asked her if she tried to convince others that she is not a witch. She said she could not do it by herself, but had the support of the ritual expert at the village who had declared that she was not a witch. What happened then that she was brought to the village? A young child died in the village and she was accused of causing the death of that child. After a short discussion with the interpreter, she gave us further details, to indicate that she thinks the death of the child was caused by something else and she suspected that it was malnutrition. When the child was born, she said she did not grow well and at the time when the child would have been crawling around, that did not happen because the child did not have enough food to eat. To the surprise of everyone, the mother was already pregnant. Since there was not enough to feed the child with, that child died. She specifically said through the interpreter, the child died for lack of food. This conversation opened a window into the broader dialogue about misfortune. Not all people think misfortune is caused by witches. In this case the victim thought the parents had neglected their own child and then turned around and blamed someone else, and in a context where many feared the alleged powers of witches, no one asked any questions.

This account clearly demonstrated to us why a pluralistic approach to the question of witchcraft is important. In her own mind, Rosemary and other villagers knew that the baby did not have food and although she did not express it that way, the child had developmental problems because of malnutrition which eventually took his life. No one knows the economic circumstances of the parents of the child, but one could also raise questions regarding spacing of children and birth control. The fact that the mother was already pregnant with another child (at a time when villagers expected her to wait until her baby started crawling) indicates that child and maternal health concerns continue to be issues that need to be addressed to reduce illnesses which are blamed on others who are then accused of being witches.

When the medical team finally arrived in Gnani in June of 2015, two male sibling children (approximately 3 and 6 years-old) were presented for treatment that were severely malnourished and needed immediate medical intervention. (See "Malnutrition" Photo 4.1.) The couple did not seem overly concerned about the fate of the children who were dressed in rags—one so weak he could not hold up his head and the other unable to sit upright. The couple was more concerned about their own medication than with their children's welfare, and they were quite reticent to work with the medical team to transport the children for acute pediatric care and critical laboratory/diagnostic testing. The medical team insisted that the children receive care. The next morning, the team purchased new clothing and diapers, bathed the children to bring their high temperatures down and clean them, and transported the children two hours to Tamale Regional Hospital. Locals had a good knowledge of these issues with the children. They may not have been overtly judgmental, but the kind of "social distance" we witnessed the other villagers keep from this couple was telling.

Chapter Three

Medical Concepts of Disease and Interpretations of Illness

We will now place witchcraft in a broader context when we examine biological mechanisms and medical concepts of disease and illness, introducing biomedical concepts in an attempt to further examine local Ghanaian, African, and Western etiologies of disease. We will then expand this situational context by examining the states of urban and rural health systems in Ghana to understand the two paradigms of healing, access, and capabilities to treat illnesses and diseases. What follows will be a contemporary discourse of endemic diseases—and their probable associations to witchcraft indictments—such as: communicable diseases (HIV/AIDS, TB, and Leprosy); malaria; epilepsy and seizures; albinism; mental illnesses; the curse of multiple births; and vision care challenges.

When we review the history of medicine, we must realize and admit that it has only been in the last 300 years—compared to the balance of humanity—that the "Germ Theory of Disease" has come about. Many of these villages exhibit ancient lifestyles with little contact with the outside world, living in thatched mud huts, just as their ancestors have been doing for generations with no running water or electricity. For them, the "Germ Theory of Disease" is a completely irrelevant and foreign idea. This unspeakably hard and challenging life in northern Ghana marked by underdevelopment and a desire to lay blame is unsatisfied by explaining the disease as caused by a mosquito bite (via invisible and deadly parasites) robbing one family of a cherished child while rather inexplicably sparing the life of another (Palmer 2010, 2). The idiosyncratic Western-world's concept that a miniscule germ (that you can't even see) can strike down a vibrant healthy human being is complicated to explain, and even more difficult to defend to a (non-medical) layperson. Since belief in witchcraft is passed down from generation to generation from the time of infancy, it is easy to understand the difficult challenge it is to get them to give up these beliefs. In fact, the history of Western medicine is filled with its own instances of prolonged resistance to changing their ideas even in the face of incontrovertible evidence. Therefore, when we are cognizant of our own historical past, we must remember to approach other cultures' theories with integrity and humility.

We can begin our journey by reviewing puerperal fever, which leveled a huge toll on maternal mortality in Europe in the seventeenth and eighteenth centuries. "Epidemics of puerperal fever are to women what war is to men. Like war, they cut down the healthiest, bravest and most essential part of the population: Like war, they strike their victims in the prime of their lives," explained Jacques-Francois-Edouard Hervieux (Dobson 2008, 74). Interestingly, around that same time, Dr. Ignaz Semmelweis, a Hungarian physician, was working in Vienna's famous teaching hospital, Allgemeines Krakenhaus. There were two obstetrical clinics in the Austrian hospital. Expectant mothers were randomly allocated to either clinic. One of the clinics was run for and by midwives in training, and the other clinic (where Semmelweis worked) was used solely for the training of medical students. During that era, it was not uncommon for a medical student or physician to move directly from performing an autopsy to delivering a baby—without changing clothing, donning gloves, or performing even a rudimentary handwashing. In 1846 Dr. Semmelweis had a colleague, a professor of forensic medicine, develop an acute infection and die after cutting his finger during an autopsy. Semmelweis also noticed that the occurrence of puerperal fever was much higher in the ward run by medical students than the ward for the midwives who performed no autopsies. He instituted a handwashing policy with a somewhat caustic mixture of chloride of lime and the incidence of puerperal fever fell dramatically. He was not terribly popular amongst his peers however, and shortly after he left, they quickly abandoned his unpopular handwashing regimen. The puerperal fever incidence then shot back up; the doctor was to later die, unheeded and disbelieved, in an insane asylum. After his death, with the findings of Pasteur and Lister gaining popularity, Semmelweis' findings were again to be "rediscovered" (Dobson 2008, 76), even though his findings predated both by some 20 years. Historically, it would prove impossible to calculate how many women died due to doctors who couldn't be bothered to wash their hands. Therefore it is with limitless gratitude and profound humility that we write today about medicine's past and current diseases and the indigenous beliefs that continue to shroud, mystify, and encompass them.

Before we move on to consider specific diseases, let us briefly examine the belief systems as to the causes of various diseases indigenous to Africa. Unfortunately we were unable to locate a typology specific to Ghana; however G.P. Murdock created such an ethnographic typology after studying 139 randomly selected societies of the world, with 43 of them located in Africa (Green 1999). His major divisions were natural vs. supernatural theories of illness causation. More recently the term "natural" has been replaced by "impersonal," and "supernatural" by "personalistic." A "personalistic" medical system is one in which illness is explained as due to the active purposeful intervention of an agent. The agent may be human (as in a sorcerer or witch) or non-human (as in an ancestor, ghost, evil spirit, or deity), and the sick person is a victim of aggression or punishment directed only at themselves. Many anthropologists characterize native African health beliefs as operating mainly in the domain of witchcraft, sorcery, or spirits (Green 1999). Another distinction to consider is the concept of "immediate or proximate" cause of illness and "ultimate cause." If an illness were considered "natural," yet does not respond to the customary treatment, then another "personalistic or ultimate" cause is suspected such as witchcraft (Green 1999, 41).

As an example, a person may have a known disease such as malaria, yet they do not respond to conventional treatments. In Western medicine, we look for explanations of this variability in treatment response by considering differing virulence of causative agent and host variations in immunity and defense. We also consider the impact of other chronic medical conditions such as diabetes, HIV, or malnutrition, which may have a deleterious effect on a patient's immune system and their ability to fight off infection and/or recover from a disease. In the witchcraft model the fact that he doesn't respond to treatment or dies (when others recover) may be attributed to a curse or spiritual retribution for violation of a taboo. Even if a man falls from a tree and injures himself, he immediately suspects another person or spirit as being the ultimate cause (Dobson 2007). In this way a kind of coexistence of scientific theories of illness and indigenous beliefs occurs. The treatment of a Western physician may be accepted, but they also consult the local spiritual healer. Africans are practical in this way; why take chances after all?

Now let us examine these concepts utilizing a hypothetical case: A young woman has died and the leaders of the village in remote, rural Ghana have come together to investigate why. What were the medical details of her death? Did she contract Malaria, meningitis, consume polluted water, or die due to some undiagnosed congenital defect? In some rural northern areas in Ghana, it just doesn't seem to matter; seemingly someone is to blame. Furthermore, oftentimes even if professional healthcare providers and medical laboratories identify a compelling medical cause—either while the "spellbound" or "cursed" victim is ill or posthumously—nevertheless someone can be blamed for cursing the person so that they caught the disease. Therefore, in many Ghanaian convictions these two major causal structures—magic and Germ Theory—are intricately intertwined, forming a belief system that creates both the potential and presage for "sending sickness" and contracting "jealousy sickness" (Farmer 1990, 21). This "medical pluralism" combines healing concepts from Western pharmaceuticals, plants, Islamic medicines, biopower, magic, and more. As Robson explains: "the pluralistic medical culture of the Dagomba" dictates no official institutions or "gatekeepers" (such as professionally licensed physicians), but rather "everybody diagnoses and everybody treats illnesses," so no one is held to be the singular "expert" in medicine (2007, 86–87). As Western medical healthcare providers, we stand squarely at the crux of this dilemma; powerless to "explain away" diseases, illnesses, and deaths owing to pathological geneses.

Let us now examine Western medical explanations of disease in order to define some of dissimilarities in fundamental beliefs. In our hypothetical example of the unexpected death of the young man, what mechanisms are used to investigate the causes and why? First of all, in most instances in such a tragedy, the victim would likely have been brought to an emergency department at their local area hospital where healthcare professionals would attempt to diagnose potential cause(s) and resuscitate (if possible). If the patient is brought in DOA (dead on arrival) or dies in the emergency department, the local coroner would be contacted, and in most cases an autopsy is performed by a trained pathologist (a doctor who specializes in the causes and effects on the body of disease or damage). The corpse would be dissected, and blood and body fluid samples obtained for culture and toxicological evaluation, and (eventually) a cause of death would be determined, recorded and reported. Once a cause of death is determined, the family is notified, and if questionable ("foul play") was involved, law enforcement officials are contacted for further criminal investigation.

The basis of our system is science; but where does this foundation originate? What it all comes down to is how we determine "truth?" The basis of modern-day "truths" in rural Ghana are that witchcraft is woven into the everyday fabric of their lives and when something bad happens someone is to blame. Conversely, as Western medical practitioners, we believe in the Germ Theory of Infection, that things we eat and habits we have can cause disease. We also believe in genetic disorders that lead to disease, and that bad things happen to good people. We don't look for someone to blame unless there is forensic "evidence" that supports it. Then whether it is a crime or medical malpractice or an accident we believe that 'evidence' must be proven in a court of law before blame can be placed on someone. However, the system was not always like that, and we will explore later on (in chapter 3.1 "American Witchcraft under Scientific Scrutiny") that the fear of witchcraft was once an integral part of the beliefs of both our American and European ancestors.

Misinformation and dogmatic beliefs were taught to countless physicians for a thousand years based on erroneous observations by men such as Galen and others who were revered until the scientific revolution destroyed these beliefs and discovered the truth. Our modern scientific method was born in an age in Europe that was dominated originally by the Roman Catholic Church. Any scientific discoveries that brought about conclusions that were contrary to the doctrine of the church would be met with reprisals and persecutions from the church. For instance, Galileo, a noted Italian scientist, spent the last years of his life under house arrest by the church for concluding that the earth revolved around the sun. Until Cartesian "dualism," the proposal was that the mind is an immaterial substance distinct from body (Crane 2000) which allowed for the mind and soul to be the realm of the church, and allowed that the 'separate body' could be the purview of medicine. Hence the metaphysical mind and soul then became the purview of the church, and scientists were able to start experimenting on the physical body.

Prior to the scientific method, there was debate between rationalists and empiricists on how to determine what was considered "truth." Rationalists essentially believed that all truth stemmed from logic, and one should be able to determine truth by using pure logic (if this is true then logically that must be true, and so on). A rationalist did not require any supporting evidence that their logic was "true." To a rationalist, logic is king and experiments are not necessary. On the other hand, empiricists only believed in "truths" made evident by sensory experience and/or evidence (particularly corporeal knowledge) in the development of theory—rather than the perception of inherent traditions or concepts.

Modern scientific theory emanates from empiricism and this has led to the scientific method of today. The medicine we practice is increasingly becoming more scientific with the modern examination of everything we perform using "evidence-based medicine," which has been defined as "the conscientious, explicit and judicious use of current best evidence in making decisions about the care of individual patients" (Sackett 1996, 71). The practice of evidence-based medicine means integrating individual clinical expertise with the best available external clinical evidence from systematic research (Sackett 1996). While all of modern medicine has some basis in science, much of what we do has come from traditional methods (hence "it's always been done that way"). However, in the early 1990s physicians began to examine everything through the lens of empirical science and research—from drug dosages to Cardio-Pulmonary Resuscitation (CPR). Since then, many changes have occurred due to this movement to "question" every technique and belief, and thereby, help eradicate dogma. Hence, in modern Western medicine, empiricism reigns supreme.

That being said, Western medicine in America suffers many "pains" as an imperfect healthcare system. American physician, self-proclaimed social revolutionary and one-man show, Dr. Hunter "Patch" Adams voices a unique and positive approach to health and healing, claiming that American healthcare is too costly, dehumanizing, mistrustful, grim, and more like an expensive business transaction rather than a holistic (whole body-mind) service-oriented caregiver-patient relationship (Adams 1993). Dr. Adams, who makes house calls and spends up to four hours taking each patient's initial history, explained that the American medical system struggles under many ills, including: poor "bedside manner" patient-doctor communications (too impersonal and hurried); provider "burnout" due to imbalanced work and personal lives; operating as a business deal (rather than a cooperative patient-doctor effort) which leads to stress and distrust; and "saddest of all, the malpractice climate denies the physician the right to be imperfect" (Adams 1993, 32). Additionally, any two cultures can clash, misinterpret, and misjudge one another when they come into contact. Barriers of language translations, customs, *Weltanschauung* ("world outlook"), ethos, and expectations for healthcare treatment can all hinder and hamstring interactions between healthcare provider and patient. In Anne Fadiman's book *The Spirit Catches You and You Fall Down: A Hmong Child, Her American Doctors, and the Collision of Two Cultures*, the author explores the lack of understanding between American healthcare staffers and a young Hmong refugee child with severe epilepsy. Some of the American's "healing practices" such as blood sampling, asking personal questions about the patient, undressing the patient, not treating the patient's soul (only the body), not knowing an immediate diagnosis/cause of illness (instead waiting days for x-ray and laboratory test results) and the removal and or cutting of the human body and its organs—ran directly in opposition to the Hmong's healing customs. As the author notes, "One doctor called them 'collisions,' which made it sound as if two different kinds of people had rammed into each other, head on, to the accompaniment of squealing brakes and breaking glass," however these encounters were "messy but rarely frontal. Both sides were wounded, but neither side seemed to know what had hit it or how to avoid another crash" (Fadiman 1997, viii). This strikes us as a fitting analogy between the colliding worlds and cultural gaps between Western medicine and Ghanaian witchcraft's healing convictions.

Therefore, when we write about the care available to people who are removed from centers of scientific practice and who live in poverty, we must recognize that much of the nation lives in a very modern, contemporary world. In Ghana, there is a dichotomy that practically comprises physical boundaries. The closer you are to the coast (the Gulf of Guinea), the more populous cities, and industry—the more modern life is, including electricity, running water, and relatively up-to-date hospitals and schools. In the far north, where we served in our clinics, these people are living a provisional life of extreme hardship, much as they have for hundreds of years. Many contemporary Ghanaians have never traveled to the northern regions of Ghana, and have little understanding (or compelling interests) that motivate them to be involved or affected by the underprivileged and marginalized day-to-day lives of these isolated villagers.

The government of Ghana has an active and effective Ministry of Health and they started a national health insurance scheme in 2003 meant to provide low cost health insurance eventually on a universal basis. It requires a buy-in that is very low cost and is supposed to cover many illnesses and situations including emergency care. Unfortunately, it has some very serious problems and in 2012 a WHO report noted that it was felt to be inadequately financed and threatening to go insolvent in 2013 (WHO 2012). Last summer when we visited, the problem of nonpayment of physicians in the insurance scheme for services rendered was causing a lot of consternation among physicians and nurse midwives who hadn't been paid for many months.

The benefit package of the NHIS consists of basic healthcare services, including outpatient consultations, essential drug(s), inpatient care (shared accommodation), maternity care (normal and caesarean delivery), eye, dental, and emergency care. After reviewing the coverage(s), we can surmise that approximately 95 percent of most diseases and illnesses are covered under Ghanaian NHIS. Nevertheless, some services classified to be elective (discretionary and/or non-compulsory), or very high-priced are listed on NHIS' exclusion list. Among these excluded services and drugs are: cosmetic surgery, drugs not listed on the NHIS drugs list (including antiretroviral drugs), cancer care, assisted reproduction, organ transplantation, private inpatient accommodation, and others.

AMERICAN WITCHCRAFT UNDER SCIENTIFIC SCRUTINY

The days of the notorious seventeenth-century American Salem witch trials—observed as the worst outbreak of witch persecution in American history—have yet to be socially and scientifically resolved even in our current twenty-first century. The infamous American Salem witch trials began in 1692, after a group of young girls in Salem Village in New England, Massachusetts, claimed they were possessed by Satan. Rampant fear and hysteria among the Puritans led to widespread panic of suspected witchcraft allegations. In May of 1692, special courts of Oyer (to hear) and Terminer (to decide) were created to hear witchcraft cases for several counties in Massachusetts. During the infamous 1692–1693 trials, over 200 people were accused of practicing witchcraft and approximately 37 were killed or died (historical numbers vary). Though the Massachusetts General Court was to annul the guilty verdicts, bitterness lingered, and the disturbing legacy of the witch trials was to endure in the collective American psyche for centuries. Every American student learns about Salem in elementary school; American children and adults alike dub any unjust persecution of a specified enemy (with no regard for his/her guilt or innocence) in the court of public opinion as a "witch hunt."

Any complete understanding of the Salem witchcraft accusations must also attempt to explain why the vast majority of accused witches were women. Carol Karlsen included Salem Possessed in her critique of histories of Salem which, "note that witches were usually women, most works pass over the fact quickly or conclude that witches were scapegoats for hostilities and tensions that had little to do with sex or gender." Although the directions the accusations took undoubtedly reflected pre-existing tensions within the community, Karlsen argues that the accusations also reflected societal ideas about women and the ways men reconciled changes in gender roles.

The problem of the "unsolved mystery" of American-propagated witchcraft has been approached and scrutinized by a variety of disciplines: sociology, psychology, political science, medical science, history, religion, gender (women's) studies, anthropology, government institutions, and legal (civil and criminal court) agencies, just to name a few. But can medical science elucidate, or perhaps even solve, these Salem witch trails? In fact, some modern-day scientific studies are now pointing to unrecognized (biologically driven) health crises as potential catalyst(s) for the (socially enforced) hysteria. One such study is Linnda Caporael's 1976 epidemiological inquiry, which pointed to the plausible widespread consumption of ergot, a poisonous fungus that grows on rye in cool, damp weather, and is the chemical source of the psychedelic drug lysergic acid diethylamide, or LSD. Among the symptoms of severe ergotism is spasms of limbs, tongue, and facial muscles, epileptic seizures, partial paralysis, coma, formication (a feeling that ants are crawling under the skin), and death; 24 of the 30 "bewitched" persons reported convulsions and sensations of being pinched, pricked, or bitten (Matossin 1982). Matossian goes on to explain how endemic health crises can pose biosocial enigmas: The physical, mental, and social disturbances that plagued Salem Village in 1692 were not unique to that time and place. Indeed, available evidence suggests that witchcraft accusations in 1692 in New England were prompted by an epidemic of ergotism, and that the Salem witchcraft affair may have been a largely unrecognized, but endemic, health problem in the New World according to Matossian (1982).

Not all scholars concur with Motassian's and Coprael's medical cause for the physical symptoms and social chaos. Four dissenting illustrations from varying disciplines include historians that assert psychological and somatic disorders (Edward Bever 2000), or Indian attacks coupled the presence of too many older, single women leading to a collective social panic (Marion Starkey 1969), or violent and intense factionalism (Paul Boyer and Stephen Nissembaum 1974), and finally psychologists N.K. Spanos and Jack Gottlieb (1976) assert a social, not physiological, explanation. Other divergent medical causes such as encephalitis, Huntington's disease, psychosomatic disorders, PTSD, Lyme Disease, and Artic Hysteria (pibloktoq) have been investigated by Laurie Winn Carlson, Anne Zeller and others (Layhew 2013).

Witchcraft researchers like Zeller, Boyer, Caporael, Matossian, and Nissenbaum not only enable us to grasp the outbreak of accusations in Salem as part of an endemic health issue or a larger pattern of communal conflict—but perhaps more notably (and ominously) serve as a cautionary tale of how acrimonious and discriminatory powers can wield, incite, and instigate modern-day witch hunts.

STATE OF URBAN VS. RURAL HEALTHCARE IN GHANA

Ghana's population as of 2010 was approximately 24,648,823, with the life expectancy improving in the last 10 years from about 58 to 63 years of age. The disease profile in Ghana is evolving as changes in availability of medical care, and improved ability to treat many infectious diseases causes people to live longer and survive to develop more degenerative non-infectious diseases such as hypertension, stroke, heart disease, and cancer. Additionally, as the infrastructure of roads and availability of motor vehicles expands, so too does the impact of traumatic injuries and deaths from motor vehicle accidents.

This is reflected in the statistics reported to the WHO which is broken down in terms of communicable, non-communicable diseases (NCDs) and trauma. At the present time the largest of all of these categories of maladies is communicable diseases at 52 percent, followed by NCDs at 41 percent, and injuries and accidents at 7 percent. Over the next 20 years they expect communicable disease to drop to 40 percent, NCDs to increase to 47 percent, and trauma to increase to 14 percent (WHO 2012). The main causes of childhood disease and death are malaria, diarrhea, respiratory infections, and neonatal conditions; while adult mortalities are attributed to HIV, hypertension, diabetes, and traffic accidents (WHO 2012). Our experience at the Gnani witches' villages echoes this finding with the most patients being treated clinically for malaria, respiratory infections, diarrheal illness, and skin diseases. We also noted cases of extremely elevated blood pressure in many of the adults.

Nonetheless, as we have pointed out, the Ghanaian Health Service has been undergoing a major transition from a "cash-and-carry" system to the National Health Insurance Scheme (NHIS) (which was adopted in 2003) and officially enacted in 2005. The system was created to remove financial barriers to health care, attempting to remove point-of-service fees, making health care affordable while improving access and healthcare outcomes. It is organized by districts (as geographical areas), with each district administering the NHIS. There are also provisions for private insurance schemes. Apparently for formal sector workers, membership is mandatory in either the NHIS or a private insurance scheme, however the majority of the population is made up of 'informal workers' who are required to pay a fee to join (based on a sliding scale according to their ability to pay) from approximately 7.2 Cedis to 48 Cedis. There is a six-month gap between joining and becoming eligible for benefits (Brugiavini and Pace 2010). However, there are some patients who are exempt from these charges. District Health Insurance Committees are tasked with identifying and categorizing residents into four main social groups: the core poor (indigent), the poor, the middle class, and the wealthy. The core poor, together with Social Security and National Interest Trust pensioners (SSNIT) over 70 years old, and children under 18 (if/when both parents pay their premiums) are exempted from paying any premium. The rest of the funding for the NHIS comes from 2.5 percent deduction from the paychecks of the formal sector workers, with some 2.5 percent of the VAT is designated to the NHIS (Brugiavini and Pace 2010). The NHIS is administered by officials in each district and paid for by subsidies from the national government. Each 'district scheme' must provide a minimum package of services that is quite comprehensive. Services that are covered include: general outpatient and inpatient services at accredited facilities, oral health, eye care, emergencies, and maternity care (prenatal care, normal delivery and some complicated deliveries). Still it is disturbing to note that HIV antiretroviral treatment and cancer treatment are not covered (Brugiavini and Pace 2010).

The majority of healthcare in Ghana is provided by the government and managed by the Ministry of Health and the Ghana Health Service. The government healthcare system has five primary tiers of care: health posts (first-level primary care for rural areas); health centers and clinics; district hospitals; regional hospitals; and tertiary hospitals. According to a 2013 news article, as many as 13 percent of these facilities have no physicians staffing them, only nurses and other healthcare community staffers (Lassey et al. 2013). There are also hospitals and clinics run by the Christian Health Association Ghana. Healthcare availability is much better in urban areas, while rural areas are understaffed, and lack proper supplies and equipment. Patients in these rural areas must either travel long distances for care, or resort to traditional health care practitioners.

All of this is well and good, except it depends on satisfactory fulfillment of the obligations NHIS accrues when card-holders present for services. Ever since its inception (despite a published policy that claims should be reimbursed within 4 weeks of filing), there have been substantial delays in payment. There have been problems of inadequate funding of the service, as well as confusion in the filing of claims, which have led to these delays.

In many cases hospitals have had problems being able to purchase supplies and medicines necessary to provide care and keep the doors open. Apparently in recent years, both hospitals and providers (physicians and nurse-midwives who are supposed to accept NHIS insurance) have started requiring cash payments from NHIS cardholders. This problem has become so serious that the National Health Service issued a directive to healthcare facilities to not turn away NHIS cardholders (Osam 2015). Another perceived problem is the abuse of the healthcare system by cardholders. They apparently come to the clinic for minor ailments, attempt to get medical treatment for uninsured relatives, and even furnish their insurance cards to their (uninsured) relatives.

As a medical team ourselves, we have run head-on into the national 'cash-and-carry' system. One of our young patients, Zebedee, (who was about to have his leg amputated from a severe infection) didn't have NHIS. Since there is a six-month lag between applying for coverage and having coverage, his surgical and treatment was cash only. World Missions Possible had to pay for everything in advance before anything—including an x-ray or exam—would be done to help Zebedee. Many long-distance phone calls later, Flowers persuaded a surgeon in Tamale to try and save the child's leg—but the surgeon and the hospital only helped the boy after all funds were secured in their accounts. Zebedee, now fully recovered, is a joyful young man who happily runs to school—on both legs.

Yet perhaps the most significant challenge to Ghanaian health care is the lack of health care providers in the country. When we first began our medical outreaches to Ghana in 2007 there were approximately 2,600 physicians in the country with most of them living and working in urban areas. Ghanaian medicine has been the victim of a substantial "brain drain." Many of the graduates from Ghanaian medical schools were drawn away to other countries in Africa as well as the United States, Great Britain, Australia, etc., where they could emigrate and make a substantially more lucrative living. At the same time there were estimated to be less than 800 Ghanaian physicians living and working in the United States and United Kingdom (Groenhout 2012). While this represents a miniscule proportion of the physicians in these two developed countries, if they had stayed in Ghana, the physician workforce would be expanded by around 30 percent. Physician density reports show that in Ghana there is 1 physician per 10,000 people (a 1:10,000 ratio) compared with the United States, where there is 1 physician per 408 people (a 1:408 ratio), or France where there is 1 physician per 319 people (1:319 ratio) (CIA 2015).

This leaves a huge deficit in available healthcare providers in the country but even more so in the remote regions. For instance at Yendi Government Hospital (the nearest large facility to Gnani), we found (usually) only one Ghanaian physician and a visiting surgeon from Cuba. There were also some nurse-midwives for delivering babies, but nearly all of the routine care was facilitated by nurses, with little physician supervision, except in acute and/or surgical cases.

With all of the problems of the NHIS, the general public of Ghana at least has certain care options. However, the healthcare options available to condemned witches, in remote regions such as the witches' village, are even more limited. They are socially feared and/or shunned, live in extreme poverty (with no means to pay for the NHIS), are without transportation, and so on and so forth. According to the policy, they should qualify as 'core poor' and be exempt from paying for NHIS coverage—but with no one to assist the Gnani residents to sign up, it is improbable that they will seek and receive access to proper care.

ENDEMIC DISEASES AND ILLNESSES

The original catalyst or "moment of epiphany" that linked our "Western medical world" to "Gnani's witches world" occurred back in 2007. The medical team was treating an elderly woman who had a horrible, open wound on her ankle, exposed all the way to the bone. Instead of helping her receive treatment for this infected wound (which had become osteomyelitis) she had been accused of sacrificing her skin in pagan ceremonies by her brother and his servant, and was summarily exiled to Gnani. Our medical team provided wound care and oral antibiotics, but we were new to the northern region (back in 2007), and were unsuccessful in locating anyone who would agree to bring her food during her stay at local hospital (see figure 3.1). Our medical team was to witness firsthand her, and many others, whose unfortunate medical conditions solicited false 'social diagnoses'—scientifically erroneous interpretations of disease and illness—as witchcraft, black *juju*, spells, and demonic possessions.

Modern science can be taught to explain the germ theory of disease revealing the causes of diseases like malaria, tuberculosis, leprosy, and HIV/AIDS. Inherited diseases such as Sickle Cell Disease and albinism as well as diabetes and seizures can be treated for what they are instead. Therefore some witchcraft accusations can be linked and scientifically interpreted via disease-prone seasons in northern Ghana. The dry season (September to January) ushers in habitually high cases of Cerebral Spinal Meningitis, Guinea Worm and food poisoning, and is also characteristically an inactive period of farm work—suggesting that "one of the causes of witchcraft accusations could be idleness" (Ter Haar 2007, 79). Conversely, during the busy farming and rainy season in Ghana, the subsequent high incidence of Malaria is "often attributed to witchcraft" (Ter Haar 2007, 79).

Communicable Diseases—Leprosy, TB, and HIV/AIDS

Normally when we are working in one of the clinics, the patients waiting will crowd around sometimes so close that you are unable to even hear yourself

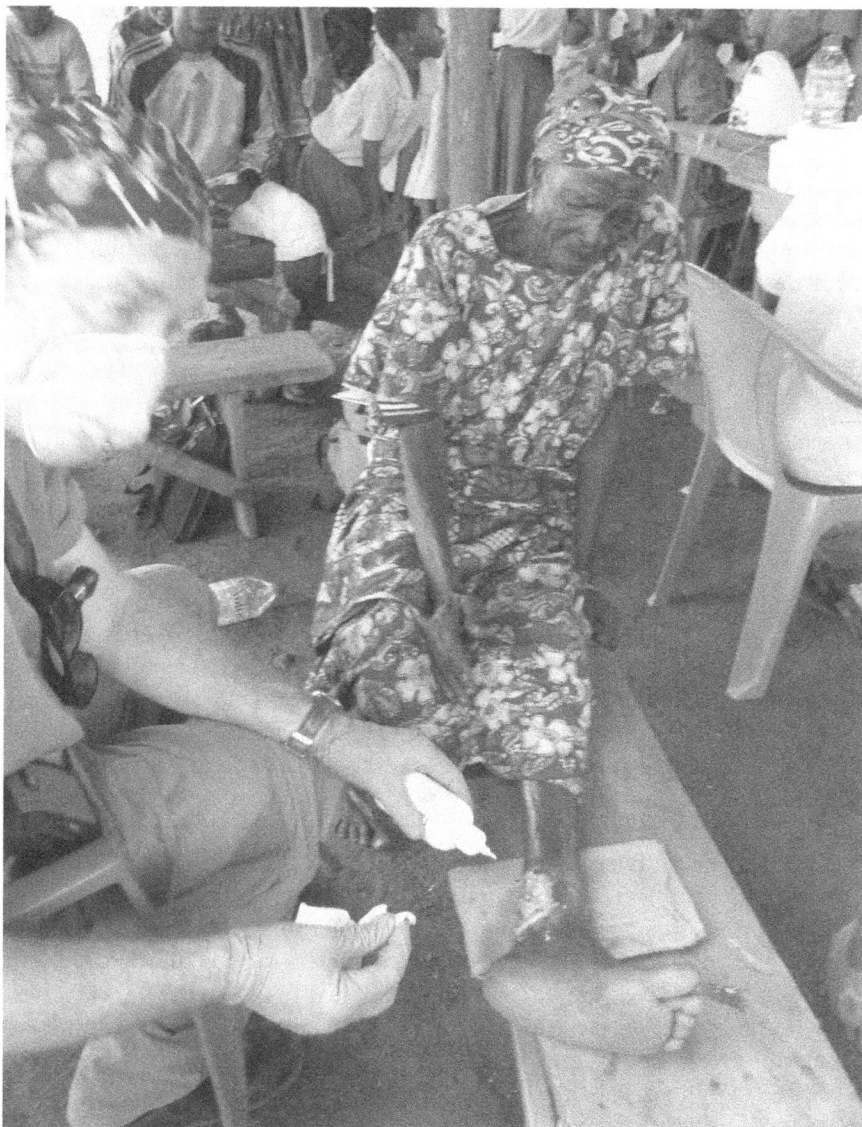

Figure 3.1.   In 2007, Drs. Flowers and Richter witness their first case of Osteo-myelitis that has a Konkomba widow condemned as a witch—she explained she was convicted of "cutting off her skin" for use in a nighttime juju ceremony.

think (much less hear any accurate sounds from your stethoscope). When we are lucky enough to be in a building, we get some relief from the clamorous din, but the doorways and windows are always jammed full with the faces of giggling children, or people attempting to be "next" in line. In 2006, as usual, news of our arrival had garnered a large crowd, perhaps around 250 people that thronged around the front and back doors of the Lawra Orphan and AIDS Centre in the Upper West region. Everyone seemed to be yelling and/or arguing, trying to jockey for a better position to get in the door. It was very hot, and the front door to the Centre was somehow always left slightly ajar, with desperate faces pressed into the tiny opening. The clinic proceeded typically, serving about 175 patients in two days.

But it was on the second day of the clinic that Richter, working triage and patient intake, noticed that—to her surprise—the doorway and hallway were both suddenly completely silent and devoid of patients. I think it was the silence that made her look up. But she didn't notice anyone standing in the doorway. Standing up from the triage desk, Richter witnessed the most pitiable sight she had ever witnessed in her numerous years working with non-profits in developing nations. In that doorway was a frail, malnourished skeleton of a man, sitting on the dusty floor in the doorway. His eyes, dulled by malnutrition, seemed more resigned than desperate—as though he was expecting, yet again, to be shunned and driven away. His clothing was threadbare and filthy, and he couldn't have weighed more than 85 pounds on his emaciated, but rather tall, frame. When you looked closely, you could see that both of his feet, part of his nose, and several of his fingers were missing. He had terrible open wounds all over the bottoms of the stumps that once held his feet. Even at first glance, it was clearly leprosy, that unspeakable, but easily diagnosed and treatable, disease. In all of her 15 years of service, Richter had never once cried in front of a patient, but it was hard to stay composed when he crawled around on the floor, refusing to sit in a chair—only asking that he get a cup of lukewarm water to stave off his thirst from crawling on his buttocks and hands for 2 kilometers to reach the WMP clinic. His name was Patrick, and after Flowers treated his wounds, he was given clean clothes, food, and a trip to the local hospital where WMP paid for his six-month treatment of antibiotics. Patrick, at age 33, had two sisters who lived in his village, but they, like all of the other villagers, were too frightened to come near him even to fetch him water from the river. That afternoon, the WMP team was unable to eat their lunch, and some gave themselves over to tears. To see such human suffering changes how you see yourself, your world, and your place in it.

However in the following year, in 2007, Patrick was unrecognizable to the WMP team as the healthy man—who slowly, but rather proudly, walked up to the WMP team, aided only by a single cane. For a mere $50—not even the cost of two music CDs—Patrick had been treated, fed, and healed of this detestable and contagious disease. He now walks easily in custom-made orthotic shoes provided by WMP in 2008, dresses in a stylish and clean suit, and is frequently visited by his friends, family members, and pastor.

In Western medicine, we know that leprosy is caused by an infection with an organism called *Mycobactrium Leprae*, which is closely related to Mycobacterium Tuberculosis. While these are both serious diseases, there are straightforward and efficacious medical treatments for both diseases. In fact in Ghana they have a specific program to treat both diseases free to their citizens. According to Atlanta-based Center for Disease Control (CDC), Leprosy (also known as Hansen's Disease) is spread person to person, most likely from coughing and sneezing (droplet inhalation). In the USA cases of leprosy do occur, primarily associated with contact with armadillos (CDC 2013), however many people appear to be resistant to the disease. Evidence shows that 95 percent of all adults are naturally protected from the disease, even if they are exposed to the bacterium that causes leprosy (CDC 2013). Cases like Patrick's are particularly disturbing due to the needless suffering, and instead of receiving free medical care, he was considered 'cursed' and forced to beg in densely populated towns, thereby infecting additional populations. Not only was his infection progressing, he was starving to death. Our team enrolled him in the national health insurance scheme, transported him to the hospital to begin treatment, provided money to buy food, and got him started on the road to recovery. Perhaps even more importantly, we explained to the local people the precautions to take to prevent transmission, so they could feel safe being around him. We left N-95 masks (particulate filter respirators certified by the CDC that protect against airborne M. tuberculo-

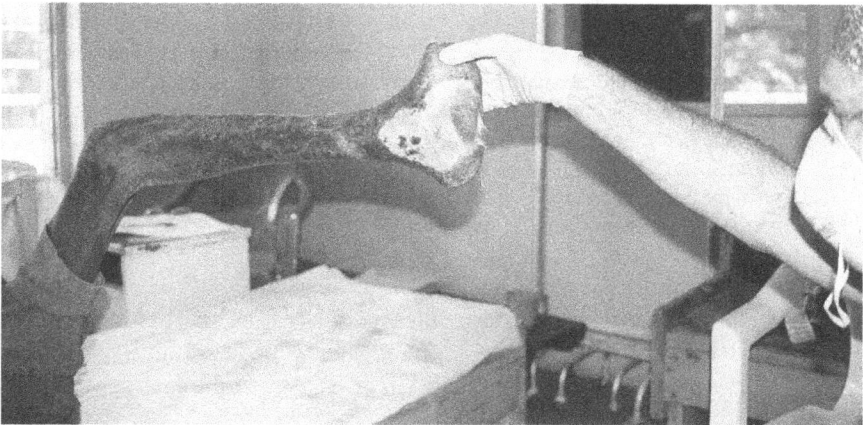

Figure 3.2.   Treating our 1st case of acute leprosy in Ghana in 2006.

sis) and nitrile ('medical grade' synthetic rubber, non-latex, puncture-resist-ant) gloves for his sisters and others who agreed to care for him. Once patients begin the appropriate leprosy therapy, the risk of transmission is exceedingly low (CDC 2013).

The problem of HIV/AIDS is yet another unique chronic, communicable disease among Gnani villagers. In Ghana, as with many other nations, there remains a significant social stigma associated with HIV/AIDS. Women in the region, in the course of prenatal care or childbirth, may be tested for HIV. If she finds out she is HIV-Positive, she may choose to conceal that diagnosis from her husband and her community for as long as possible, even though there has been a considerable push on the part of the Ghanaian Health Ser-vice to identify and make available treatment for HIV. Yet due to the stigma, many refuse to be tested and/or risk being seen taking antiretroviral therapy (ART) drugs. So extreme is the stigma that HIV-Positive women will contin-ue to breast-feed their children, even though they could pass the disease onto their children. Women in rural Ghanaian villages who choose to bottle-feed formula to their babies, as opposed to breast-feeding, run the public risk of being labeled as HIV-Positive.

These women were more concerned with the recalcitrant stigma than the health of their children. What is also even more disturbing is the prevalence in beliefs about HIV. Many of the people are suspicious of the "white peo-ple" as the cause of this disease. There is also the tragic perpetuation of counter-productive beliefs among 'natural' or traditional healers such as the "Virgin Cure." This belief is that if a man with HIV has sex with a virgin, he will be cured. This could be a virgin boy or girl and has been responsible for rapes of girls and boys at ever younger ages. In Benjamin Radford's "How Belief in Magic Spreads AIDS in Africa," the author notes in his research that:

> For many Africans even the knowledge that AIDS is caused by HIV—and that it is acquired through sexual contact—leaves room for the likelihood, or at least the possibility, that black magic caused the HIV infection in the first place. One particularly pernicious myth in Africa holds that having sex with a virgin can cure a person of AIDS. Finding treatments—and possibly even cures—for AIDS is one thing, but changing deeply-rooted cultural beliefs that perpetuate the disease is almost as difficult. (Radford 2013, 1)

In looking into this appalling travesty, we were shocked to find that similar beliefs occurred in Western cultures only a few short centuries ago. Apparently the "Virgin Cure" was thought to be a folk-cure for syphilis and other venereal diseases in Europe and Great Britain in the late seventeenth century.

Common Disease of Malaria

Without a doubt, malaria is our most common malady affecting all ages in Gnani. Interestingly, malaria is also one of the oldest recorded diseases in human history. Even though today it is largely confined to the tropical and subtropical regions of Africa, Asia and Latin America, it has ranged as far north as the Russian Arctic and as far south as Australia and Argentina (Dobson 2007). It was found all over the Mediterranean countries, in Great Britain (known as Kentish Ague) and even the United States where it was known simply as "Ague." In the sixteenth century, the Italians were the first to call it Malaria which meant "foul air" (Dobson 2007, 86). Throughout the ages, other names for Malaria have been: Tertian Fever, Quartan Fever, Malignant Fever, Marsh Fever, Roman fever, Swamp Fever, and Blackwater Fever. Actually, it wasn't until the late nineteenth century that the cause of the disease and it's mode of transmission was discovered (Dobson 2007). Malaria is caused by the transmission to humans by the bite from an infected female Anopheles mosquito (of which there are 60 species) of one of four varieties of intra-cellular parasites known as Plasmodium Falciparum (the deadliest form), P. Vivax, P. Ovale, and P. Malariae. The parasites enter the blood stream are carried to the liver where they change into new forms that then invade the red blood cells. Every 48–72 hours (depending on the species) a cycle of multiplication is completed and the new protozoans burst from the infected red blood cells causing the periodic fevers that are the hallmark of this disease. Any other female Anopheles mosquito who bites an infected person also becomes infected and capable of spreading the disease to other humans (Dobson 2007). It is possible for the bite of one infected mosquito to cause malaria in a human being. Falciparum Malaria is the most common form found in Ghana.

Whether Malaria was present in the New World before 1492 is unclear however it is likely that early explorers and settlers from northern Europe brought Plasmodium Vivax with them to the New World. With the expansion of travel and trade between southern Europe and the advent of the slave trade brought the more deadly Plasmodium Falciparum to the Americas (Dobson 2007). Prior to the modern era and the connection with mosquitos, people in many parts of the world noticed the association with stagnant water and swamps. They felt it was from the "noxious vapors" found in marshy areas. In Africa and other regions with pronounced "rainy seasons," the disease was associated with the seasonal rains. In 1999 Ghana became part of the "Roll Back Malaria" initiative with a goal to reduce the morbidity and mortality attributed to malaria by 50 percent by the year 2010, according to the Ghana Health Service (2009). Unfortunately this goal was not achieved and a revised National Malaria Control Programme was implemented, stated the Ghana Health Service, with a revised goal of reducing deaths and illness due to malaria by 75 percent by 2015 (2009). At this time the data is still pending as to whether or not these goals have been attained. The good news is that knowledge of the cause of Malaria and its association with mosquitoes has become relatively widespread. Also there is effective treatment available in Ghana. The problems faced in these extremely rural areas is the lack of transportation to access medical care and due to the remoteness, there is suspicion of 'Western witchcraft' treatments and medical doctors—views, to some extent, perpetuated no doubt by traditional local healers and witchdoctors. There is also the coexistence of the witchcraft beliefs and the idea of an "ultimate cause" which may be witchcraft if one person dies when others recover from malaria (ITCD, 41). This would be the example in their beliefs of a person dying from a medical condition as a victim of witchcraft. Then a divination procedure as described already would be done to look for the 'witch' who caused this result.

"Demonic Possession" — Epilepsy

Similarly, it is exceedingly common for people with seizures to be condemned as witches. As such, they are believed to be possessed by demons rather than having a medical condition that needs treatment. When you consider the plight of a person with epilepsy in remote areas of Ghana it becomes an affliction in which the social stigmata can be more damaging—and limiting—than the disease itself. While it is understandable that, in a culture in which belief in supernatural causes for most afflictions is the norm, a grand mal seizure would be considered visible evidence of such a problem. We know that seizures can be the manifestation of many diseases, varying widely according to the age and condition of the patient. In 2009, at one of our clinics at Gnani, a man suffered a grand mal seizure in front of us. It was self-limited but a pastor who had traveled with us attempted to "exorcise" him of the demon causing the seizure. The man's seizures were the reason for his being exiled to the Gnani witches' village. He had never been able to be treated by a medical doctor for his condition. We have witnessed several other patients who gave a history of epilepsy.

For those who have never witnessed a grand mal seizure, it can prove to be a very shocking and rather distressing incident. The person flails around on the floor, with violent jerking of their limbs, they can scream, and even have bloody sputum 'froth' at their mouths if they bite down on their own tongue. As opposed to petite mal seizures (a.k.a., simple or complex "absence" seizures), grand mal (a.k.a., generalized tonic-clonic) seizures have two stages: tonic (first) phase is when the patient's muscles stiffen, they lose consciousness, fall to the floor, and the person can bite their tongue or cheek (bloody saliva). After the initial tonic phase comes the clonic phase when the arms and legs can jerk rapidly and rhythmically for (usually) 1 to 3 minutes.

Any seizures that last longer than 5 to10 minutes (convulsive status epilepticus) require immediate emergency care. The following signs and symptoms occur in some (but not all patients) that have grand mal seizures: a 'warning' feeling of numbness (Aura); a scream (muscles seize around the vocal cords and force air out); a loss of bowel and/or bladder control; unresponsiveness or unconsciousness after convulsing; disorientation (postictal confusion); fatigue; sleepiness; and severe headaches (Mayo Clinic 2016).

As Dr. Lowenstein explains, the condition of epilepsy can take on a myriad of symptoms and complications:

> A seizure is a paroxysmal event due to excessive or synchronous neuronal activity in the brain. Depending on the distribution of the discharges, this abnormal brain activity can have various manifestations ranging from dramatic convulsive activity to experiential phenomena not readily discernible by an observer. Epilepsy describes a condition in which a person has recurrent seizures due to a chronic, underlying process. There are many causes and forms of epilepsy. (Lowenstein 2011, 3251)

But it is not only epilepsy that can cause people to suffer from seizures. The medical list of diseases with seizures as a part of their symptomatology is extensive and includes the following categories: infectious processes, febrile seizures, traumatic lesions, toxic conditions, metabolic disturbances, neoplastic disease, vascular disorders, neurocutaneous disorders, neurodegenerative disorders, and other miscellaneous (Marx et al 2013). Each of these categories has multiple diagnoses—which can never be diagnosed and/or treated—if the patient is never able to seek proper medical care.

Currently, there are estimated to 50,000,000 Persons With Epilepsy (PWE) worldwide and approximately 80 percent live in developing countries, with a population ratio prevalence at approximately 5 to 10:1,000 people (Dugbartey and Barimah 2014). However, when PWE believe the cause of epilepsy to be supernatural, it would (seemingly) prove illogical to seek care at a hospital or medical clinic. Therefore, sociocultural beliefs and attitudes continue to be a tremendous barrier to treatment and a cause of discrimination and stigmatization of PWE. Rather a person unfortunate enough to suffer from periodic epileptic seizures in rural Ghana is subject to being considered "cursed," "demon-possessed," ostracized, and abused due to fears of contagions or demonic power practice. It is not a notable revelation to envision how many PWE end up condemned to a witches' village. Case in point: One recent study compiled among 173 university students in Ghana reflects this precise bias (Dugbartey and Barimah 2014). The study was done using a survey "Attitudes toward Persons with Epilepsy," or ATPE Study, and the results were compiled and then compared to published data collected in Ghana 30 years previously—reporting a mixed outcome of both good and bad news. In the early study, 28 percent of all interviewed Ghanaian students believed epilepsy was caused by witchcraft, which included 24 percent of these same students being "unsure" of the cause, but the other half (48 percent) noting that they were "sure" in their belief that witchcraft did not cause epileptic seizures (Dugbartey and Barimah 2014). In same-cited study, the later 2014 report noted there were still 24 percent of students who believed that epilepsy was caused by witchcraft, yet only 0.6 percent were "unsure" of the cause, and 74.6 percent were "sure" that epilepsy wasn't caused by witchcraft (Dugbartey and Barimah 2014). However there also continued to be a fallacious prevailing belief that epilepsy is contagious and an infectious disease. The earlier study reported that an overwhelming 78 percent believed it to be transmissible, conversely, in the later 2014 study the opposite was true, with 83.6 percent reporting that epilepsy was not contagious. As stated above, infectious diseases *may* be involved in some non-epilepsy cases, as noted in the other causes as described above. Fortunately, these two studies do show significant changes in the attitudes in university students in Ghana over the past 30 years; it also shows a noteworthy retention of inaccurate beliefs even among Ghana's most educated population(s). We can hypothesize that among the less-educated rural populace the exposure to modern twenty-first century scientific theories and evidence-based medical diagnoses is much less; therefore the retention of supernatural explanations would conceivably be higher than the findings among university students in contemporary urban areas.

Albinism

In addition to anti-witchcraft violence, albinos in Ghana and other African nations can suffer unnecessarily under certain destructive sorcery beliefs. Albinism is a rare, non-contagious, genetically inherited condition which occurs worldwide regardless of ethnicity or gender, and both the father and mother must carry the recessive gene for it to be passed on (even if they do not physically manifest the physical manifestations of albinism themselves). Albinism in Africa is relatively common, some 1:5,000 compared with 1:20,000 in Europe and the U.S.; some groups such as the Ibo in Nigeria and the Tonga in Zimbabwe comprise high rates of approximately 1:1,000 (Greaves 2014). Most commonly, albinism results in the lack of melanin pigment in the hair, skin and eyes (*oculocutaneous albinism*), causing vulnerability to sun exposure. Albinism is profoundly misjudged, both publicly and medically. The physical manifestations of African albinos are frequently the object of myths, bigotry, marginalization, and cruel exploitation—all of which cultivate their continued modern-day discrimination, persecution, marginalization, and exclusion.

In Ghana, albinos can be revered as embodiments of spirits, or they can struggle under inequitable access to employment, marital station, inheritance rights, and other forms of bigotry. The reality that Africa's albinos are, "either revered as spiritual incarnations or discriminated against because they translate into the ancestral world are not mutually exclusive," (Menes 2014) is a baffling enigma that proves mystifying to many casual Western observers. According to Joyce Gyamfi, the Brong-Ahafo Regional Coordinator of the Ghana Association of Persons with Albinism (GAPA), the term used in the Ghanaian Akan language to refer to Albinos is "derogatory" and local myths held about albinos includes that they suffered a 'premature birth'; that albinos don't use the bathroom to defecate/urinate on Fridays, and they do not die but rather "vanish" into the spiritual realm (Boateng 2015, 1).

In 2015, Atebubu (in the Atebubu/Amantin District of Brong-Ahafo Region) is denying Yussif Fatau, a 17-year-old student, residential access at Atebubu Senior High School (2015). According to the newspaper's report, it is an "abominable act in many cultures in Ghana for albinos to be enstooled or enskinned as Chiefs—even when they are supposed to be the legitimate successors," and furthermore some rural and traditional local areas "consider the existence of albinos as abominable, to the extent of banishing them" (Boateng 2015, 1). Reportedly, the child's father has sought safe housing for the young boy outside of the town's limits. Ankobeahene of Atebubu Traditional Area, Nana Owusu Gyimah, is a taboo for an albino to live at Atebubu and that the boy must leave the town, (as ordered by the local Traditional Authority) because his safety is not assured in the town. Gyimah said it would be best for Fatau's parents to take the boy to another student housing in another town, but: "If people want to insist it is his fundamental human rights to access education and stay in the town, then one day the parents would meet an empty room, without knowing who to ask or blame about the whereabouts of their son" (Boateng 2015, 1). This lightly veiled threat and publicly recorded intimidation against the child's life was clear: Voluntarily move the child out of the town, or he will be removed via malevolent means.

However in the past decade, the formerly "worthless" African albinos are fast becoming considered "priceless"—but not in a benevolent or well-intentioned way. Throughout Africa witchdoctors are consulted not only for healing diseases, but also for placing or removing curses or bringing luck in love or business. The belief and practice of using body parts for magical ritual or benefit is called *muti*. Witchdoctors and traditional healers in some African countries grind up human body parts (body parts from children are held to be particularly sought-after) and combine them with roots, herbs, seawater, and animal body parts to prepare potions that are then rubbed on the skin, ingested, or utilized in incantations. *Muti* murders are particularly brutal in that limbs, breasts, and other body parts are amputated from their living victims (as beliefs uphold that the "power" in the *muti* comes from the anguished cries of its victims). According to the United Nations a single albino body part can sell for around $600 (or about what the average person earns in one year) in Tanzania (Radford 2105), and up to $75,000 for a "complete set of albino body parts—including all four limbs, genitals, tongue, ears and nose" (Strochlic 2015) .

Hundreds of albino people have already been murdered in Tanzania, South Africa, and other African nations. Termed *"muti* murders" or "medicine murders," the South African Limpopo province alone recorded 250 *"muti*-murders" in a single year in a nation where 50 percent–90 percent of the population believe in black magic witchcraft (South Africa Today 2014). Albino body parts, especially the limbs, eyes, tongues, breasts, and genitals, are used in *muti* rituals by witchdoctors in an effort to bring about wealth and good fortune. A researcher in the *Journal of Investigative Psychology and Offender Profiling* explained the underlying belief system of *muti* this way:

> In traditional African beliefs, it is assumed that there is only a certain amount of luck in society. Each individual receives a portion of that luck. It is therefore believed that if another person is successful, then they have obtained an extra portion of luck via devious means, usually with the intervention of the supernatural. Setbacks or calamities, such as drought or illness, are signs that the natural and social order has been disturbed. One means of obtaining this extra portion of luck or restoring the natural order is through the use of strong *muti*. It is with this strong *muti* that *muti* murders are often associated. Muti made from human body parts is considered to be exceptionally powerful. . . . Just as different ingredients in a recipe are used for different purposes, certain body parts are used for particular goals. (Labuschagne 2004, 194)

Some uncovered examples of these rural and indigenous beliefs include: albino eyes can restore failing eyesight; the death of an albino can lift a curse; severed hands cause business success; genitals attract luck; albino hair woven into nets will catch fish; albino legs will cause a mine to produce gold; and having sexual intercourse with an albino will cure AIDS.

According to the Geneva, Switzerland-based Office of the United Nations High Commissioner for Human Rights (OHCHR):

> Persons with albinism are a unique group whose human rights issues have generally gone unnoticed for centuries; the result being deeply engraved stigma, discrimination and violence against them across various countries. The complexity and uniqueness of the condition means that their experiences significantly and simultaneously touch on several human rights issues including, but not limited to, discrimination based on color, discrimination based on disability, special needs in terms of access to education and enjoyment of the highest standards of health, harmful traditional practices, violence including killings and ritual attacks, trade and trafficking of body parts for witchcraft purposes, infanticide and abandonment of children. (OHCHR 2015)

These gruesome crimes underscore the atypical crossroads of supernatural beliefs, African culture, and government. At its essence, what can be considered "quaint" or "benign" traditional, social, religious, governmental, and media-promoted 'acceptance' (e.g., tolerance, endorsement, sanction, acknowledgement, tacit approval) of witchcraft can foster tangible—and even deadly—outcomes.

Without daily doses of a high-SPF sunscreen, pale-skinned Ghanaian albinos have little chance of escaping melanoma under the harsh sub-Saharan sun. According to Mel Greaves, a cell biologist at the Institute of Cancer Research in the United Kingdom, some 50 percent of Nigerian albinos had skin cancer by age 26, while 80 percent of Tanzanian albinos developed skin cancer by age 30, and (as a collective group), fewer than 10 percent of sub-Saharan albinos survive beyond age 40 (Greaves 2014). Aside from social maltreatment, albinos living in sub-Saharan Africa are affected by significant vulnerabilities in their eye structure development, optic nerves, and their exposure to bright sunlight. As the U.S.-based Vision for Tomorrow Foundation noted: "Eyes develop differently in someone with albinism, conventional treatments, such as surgery or eyeglasses, do not correct the problem," and the degree of reduced visual acuity varies greatly among these individuals (2015). Albinos tend to suffer with higher rates of light sensitivity, Strabismus (a.k.a., "lazy eye"), delayed visual maturation among infants, Nystagmus (involuntary eye movements), and poor vision (even after correction with corrective lenses) (Vision for Tomorrow Foundation 2015).

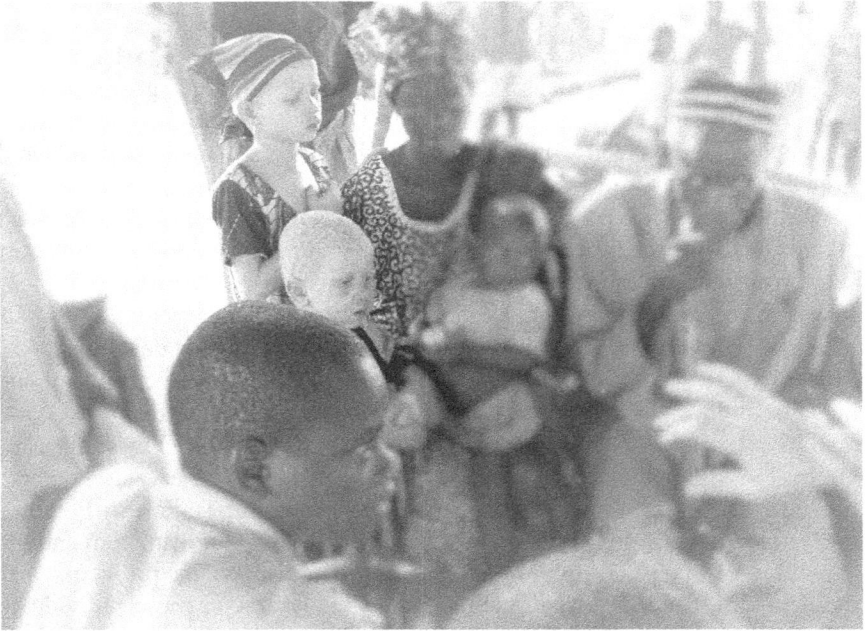

Figure 3.3. "Have the white people take the white children."

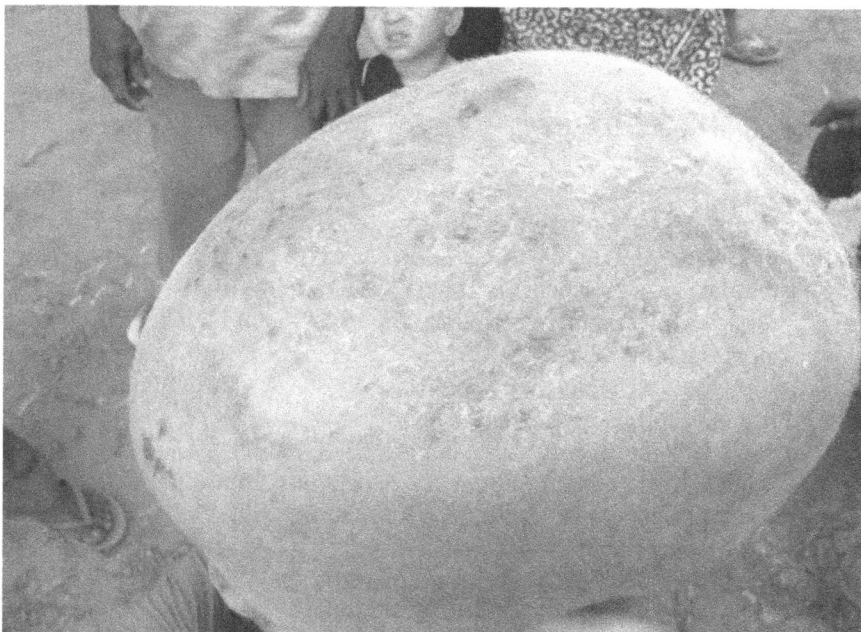

Figure 3.4. In 2008, after a post-clinic meeting with the parents, the Obroni "white people" (Flowers and Richter) realized that the parents wanted the children, but they were incessantly beaten and ostracized, so they wanted them to be safe. Already both albino children were exhibiting pre-cancerous/cancerous lesions.

We also saw some tragic cases of albinism. Scientifically we know that albinism is a genetic disease of humans which can be ocular or oculocutaneous. The ocular version only affects the pigment in the iris of the eyes and results in light blue eyes (Wolf 2005) and is predominantly seen in males. Oculocutaneous albinism affects the eyes and the skin. In the nomenclature of a geneticist, the gene for albinism is a recessive allele as compared to the genes or "alleles" for pigmented skin (there are different alleles depending on African, Asian or European descent) which are dominant. Also since the occurrence of oculocutaneous albinism has an equal occurrence between males and females, this problem isn't carried on the sex genes (these genes aren't on either the X or Y chromosome). This allows for a carrier state in which, as with the parents of these children, they appear to be normal Africans. The dominant allele is expressed. Each child will get an allele or gene from each parent. Since they are both carriers they also each have the recessive allele or gene. If you take the normal genetic grid and plot it out it will look like this: Homozygous means they have the same gene (either dominant or recessive). Heterozygous means they have a dominant gene and a recessive gene. Only the dominant gene is expressed but the person is a carrier for the recessive gene. (See "Albinism: Chart of Genetic Predictions" below.)

Hence, if both parents are heterozygous (which must be the case here), the odds of having a homozygous child with aa (albinism) is 25 percent. In other words every time this couple has a pregnancy they have a 75 percent chance of a normal appearing child (the genetic phenotypes of DD and Dr appear normal) and 25 percent chance of an albino child (phenotype rr). It is important to note that albinism itself doesn't cause any disease or mortality except through increased sensitivity and susceptibility to disease caused by sunlight. Lack of the pigment blocking ultraviolet radiation increases the risk of melanomas (skin cancers) and other problems. In physical terms, even though they look different they simply have visual problems and need protection from the sun (Boissy and Nordlund 2014).

We met with the parents after clinic one time and discovered that the children are severely ostracized and suffer beatings from other children and adults. They are also very susceptible to sunburn and skin cancer such as melanoma because their skin has no melanin for protection from the sun. Finally, they also have visual problems related to lack of melanin in the iris and problems with sensitivity to the bright sunlight. The parents of these two unfortunate children actually asked us to take their children back to the USA. They asked that the "white people" (us) take their white children. The fact that their children are albino is why they were condemned.

In a future effort to stem the ostensible rising tide of albino persecution, on 10 April of 2015, resolution A/HRC/RES/28/6 was adopted (without a vote) by the United Nations' Human Rights Council (UNHRC 2015). This resolution established a three-year segment under a mandate of UNHCR Independent Expert, Ikponwosa Ero, on the enjoyment of human rights by persons with albinism (UNHRC 2015). The resolution also recommended that Ero and her staff seek to "integrate a gender perspective throughout the work of the mandate and to pay specific attention to the challenges and needs of women and girls to address the multiple, intersecting and aggravated forms of discrimination faced by women and girls with albinism" (UNHRC 2015, 1). Additionally, a few NGOs, such as the Red Cross, the United Nations, the Ghana Association of Persons with Albinism (GAPA), and Canada-based Under the Same Sun, are attempting to protect Africans with al-

D = Dominant gene *(normal skin pigment)* *R = Recessive gene* *(for albinism)*	*D*	*r*
D	DD	Dr
r	DD	rr

binism from attacks and persecution through education, social transformation, and legislative action.

"I CARE" Vision Program

After traveling to 67 nations and conducting firsthand medical aid, disaster relief, and fieldwork outreaches in 18 nations, Richter, in her opinion, has observed and encountered three 'globally predominant gaps' in healthcare in developing nations, which include trauma/emergency care (EMS—basic and advanced trauma and cardiac life support ATLS/ACLS, and pediatric advanced life support PALS, etc.), dental care, and eye care (cataract surgery—ophthalmology; eyeglasses—optician; vision screening for glaucoma, diabetic retinopathy, corneal abrasions/ulcers, conjunctivitis, hyperopia, myopia, astigmatism, etc.—optometry). Unfortunately, only about 10 percent of people in developing nations have access to skilled eye care (Dunaway and Berger 1999). As a nonprofit, WMP primarily focuses on building Emergency Medical Services (EMS) capacities through healthcare practitioner training, materials support (CPR, trauma, and cardiac- and life-support instructions), and the donation of high-tech EMS equipment to public hospitals and clinics. Since 2009, WMP has offered free vision screening (Glaucoma, diabetic retinopathy, etc.) and eyeglasses through its "I CARE" programs in Sierra Leone, Ghana, Swaziland, and the United States (Houston, Texas). Thanks to optician Jerry Higgins, an optician, and Dr. Tom Pruett, an optometrist and co-founder of Crystal Crafters, the optical needs of WMP's Gnani patients are in not only benevolent, but experienced and skillful, professional hands. All of WMP's custom-made eyeglasses are rendered free or at-cost to our patients from Crystal Crafters, a non-profit optics lab in Lake Jackson, Texas. We are also grateful to Dr. Charles Darko-Takyi, an Optometry professor at University of Cape Coast, Ghana, who heads up our "I CARE" clinics in Ghana with the assistance of four to six of his graduating senior students. WMP receives the eyeglasses we dispense at our "I CARE" clinics from three sources: new, custom-made per patient needs, and recycled (either the frames, and one lens, or both lenses). On average, our NGO receives 1,000–2,000 donated eyeglasses per year from various nonprofit sources. Out of those donated eyeglasses, we clean the lenses, assess any scratches on the lenses, repair the frame, and/or dispose of one, both, or none of the lenses based on Pruett's set "Diopter Tolerances for Recycled Eyeglasses" formula (see Appendix). As an example, the diopter tolerance for reusing a donated pair of minus single-vision -5.50 eyeglasses would be 0.75 cylinder tolerance, and 1.00 diopter of an allowable variance between the right and left lenses. In addition to the diopter tolerances allowed under Pruett's formula, World Missions Possible also refrains from dispensing donated prescription sunglasses, bifocal, trifocal, and/or progressive lenses; pre-defined parameters of custom-only prescription eyeglasses includes all bifocal, trifocal, and high corrective astigmatisms (over 1.25 diopters or higher). World Missions Possible's rationale for using (on average) 10 percent—25 percent recycled eyeglasses (primarily reading glasses) in our "I CARE" clinics is based on Pruett's 35 years of vision care experience in developing nations. With little effort, over-the-counter reading glasses can be promptly re-used by people over the age of forty, and in an "average" adult population approximately 3.6 percent will be farsighted, 33 percent will be nearsighted, but only 3 percent will suffer from astigmatisms higher than 1.25 diopters, and about 5 percent to 15 percent of children have refractive errors (Dunaway and Berger 1999).

Pruett noted that recycled eyeglasses in rural medical outreaches are "very worthwhile" for several reasons: the fabrication of new eyeglasses for immediate delivery requires a great deal of time from skilled opticians, and even if the heavy, hard-to-transport edging equipment were to be made available/transported to a rural site—it requires both electrical power and water to function. Plus, uncut lens inventories are limited to available "stock powers," and lenses and frames (pediatric size and adult) will be limited to the number that can be transported to a site, and finally there is a significant cost factor in creating custom eyeglasses for each and every patient (Pruett 2016). However, patients are unique individuals with differing facial features and pupil distances, but fortunately there is enough symmetry between patients to allow for some "generic" fittings to serve numerous individuals. One strategic 'trick of the trade' includes using the spherical equivalent, an algebraic computation that adds half of the cylinder power to the sphere power, representing the average of the two powers that make up the spherocylinder. This is a clever equation that lets us easily compute the average power in any nonspherical lens. To explain further, a single-vision lens has refracting power of plus (+) for hyperopia or farsightedness (also used for presbyopia for people over age 40+, a.k.a., OTC 'reading glasses'), or a minus (-) for myopia or nearsightedness. Therefore a farsighted individual is hyperopic and light entering their eye is not condensed adequately to focus sharply on the retina, so they need a (+) lens to help focus light on the retina, whereas a nearsighted person's eye focuses light too soon (before it gets to his retina), so this myopic patient needs a lens to take power away, thus they need a (-) lens. Astigmatism (cylinder) errors do not focus light uniformly. So, the prescription for a person needing a visual correction can be a simple (sphere) lens or a compound (sphere and cylinder). Here are a few useful examples that will help explain spherical equivalent usage in rural fieldwork where there are no optical labs available: +1.25 is a prescription for a farsighted patient with no astigmatism; +1.25 -1.00 x 180 is a farsighted patient with astigmatism; -1.25 is a nearsighted patient with no astigmatism; and -1.25–1.00x 180 is a nearsighted person with astigmatism. Thus, the SER of +1.25 added to ½ the cylinder power of -0.50 = +0.75, and the SER of -1.25 added to ½ the cylinder power of -0.50 = -1.75. So the use of a spherical equivalent is extremely useful in rural vision-aid fieldwork as we are rarely able to manufacture custom-made eyeglasses due to a lack of equipment and/or water, so we have to rely on spherical equivalent refraction (SER) to ascertain the average power of the overall lens.

The Curse of Multiple Births

It is a complex tale to explain how, in 2006, Richter came to be crowned as *"Ama Oyemiyiefo Nksohemaa"* or "Saturday-Born Queen Mother of Compassion" in Ghana's villages of Ekotsi-Bogyano. It all had to do with Richter's support of a traditionally "taboo" set of triplets in Lawra that were born to a mentally retarded woman. It all started back in 2003 when Richter traveled to Nalerigu Baptist Medical Centre and other public hospitals to donate medical equipment through Medical Bridges, a Houston-based NGO, where she was Program Director. She met a nurse in Accra who had traveled 17 hours by bus to ask for urgent help with a set of triplets—considered a forbidden taboo—who were starving at her remote AIDS orphanage in Lawra as their severely retarded mother refused to breastfeed the three babies. The nurse explained that every set of triplets (four in total) had been killed at her orphanage as family members (usually the grandmother) would "sneak" the babies out in baskets or under their clothing in order to kill babies that "cursed" their families. The nurse stated that this set of Lawra triplets "never left her side" and were kept under 24-hour-a-day watch as the triplets' grandmother had already been caught attempting to steal the triplets from the clinic.

In seeking to understand the basis of these traditional taboos concerning multiple births (two or more) we were told two versions of this shocking taboo. The first version was that since the mother had effectively had a "litter" she must possess the spirit of a dog or a pig. The nurse from Lawra in fact explained how mothers wail, "I am not a pig!" after delivering more than two babies. The second belief is that one of the children would identify with the father, the other with the mother (this is why twins are acceptable), but the third child would "supervise" the killings of both parents. Since no one could discern which child was unlucky or doomed, one must be sacrificed (given up to be killed), or they all need to be killed. The most common method we heard about was drowning the babies (soon after birth) in the nearby lake. In the past, the mother would also be at risk to be exiled or killed along with her children. Tradition also dictates that the father of any multiple births can never look upon the children. According to the Ghana News Agency, the birth of triplets is every mother's nightmare in this northwestern region:

In communities in the Lawra District, giving birth to triplets is a taboo to their ancestral gods. Triplets are also perceived as jinxed children and it is believed that if one is not killed calamity may befall their father or the family as a whole. The Upper West Regional Multi-Sectoral Committee on Child Welfare and Protection says any woman who gives birth to triplets is given the options of offering one of them to be killed or having her husband relocated in a different community to escape the 'consequential' calamity. Mothers of triplets also stand the risk of being banished from the community should they refuse to sacrifice one of their babies. Thus having triplets in these communities is every woman's nightmare. (Pobia 2011, 1)

So in 2006, Bishop Joseph Atto Brown decided to honor Richter for her humanitarian aid in the most splendid way he could, by making her an honored Queen Mother (but usually referred to as: "*Nana*") of his village. In the native Twi language of the Akan people, "*Nana*" is a gender-neutral title representing the highest office in society, meaning grandmother, grandfather, elder(ess), venerable ancestress, and venerable ancestor. An Akan queen mother's customary responsibilities are to oversee the welfare of women in her area, and she is considered to be a wise model of motherhood with moral authority as a trusted advisor to the chief concerning community affairs. Richter's 2006 "enstoolment" was a very colorful and complex ceremony that took place during the annual Path-Clearing Festival held on the second Sunday in November. Richter was not consulted on her appointment; she was simply outfitted in a native Kente cloth and lace dress with crown and scepter—and with pomp and ceremony fit for a queen—she was seated in a special palanquin (decorated in the same Kente cloth) and in a great procession of hundreds, carried on the heads of a select group of men in a parade for about two kilometers. Some of the men carried massive, barrel-sized drums on their heads which were pounded on by other men who followed them. Suffice it to say, it was quite a spectacle, including customary local religious rituals of pouring of libations of rum. In 2007, Richter was told that this village had a grave and checkered history concerning their last Queen Mother's enstoolment ceremony in which a car had crashed into the throng of people—killing many of the villagers. Richter then was told how a Ghanaian man from town had traveled out to Richter's enstoolment ceremony in 2006—with the specific purpose of placing a witchcraft "curse" on Richter's ceremony. Seemingly, he didn't appreciate having an American *Obroni* ("white people") Christian as his Queen Mother. As he was walking along the road though, three men approached him along the road to Bogyano, and asked him what he was doing, and he told them he was on his way to place a "curse" on the ceremony and Richter. Shortly thereafter, the man was struck by a motorcycle and injured. The man never reached the ceremony as he was recuperating from his injuries. But Bishop Brown and Richter explain the story as their Christian God sending three strangers (or angels) to protect

Richter from dark omens. Since 2006, Richter has experienced several instances when Ghanaians have placed malevolent witchcraft "spells" on her: once in a bewitched "gift" of goat's milk soap (others had witnessed her stabbing pins into soap cake); and again by someone sneaking into the chief's quarters and casting spells by pouring libations over her Queen Mother's stool—which was then destroyed; and the new stool kept under lock and key.

Chapter Four

Gnani—Etiology of Diseases and Disorders

Our research's hypothesis is that some demonstrable clinical medical identification(s) in our 1,714 patient records may be one key to understanding some of these illnesses—in that a proper diagnosis by a skilled healthcare provider could alleviate some of the misconceptions that have previously led to fallacious witchcraft accusations. It is in this context that we also explore some of the health conditions, injuries, and illnesses that have been witnessed and treated at our "Clinics without Walls" such as HIV/AIDS, malaria, epilepsy, parasites, malnutrition, bacterial and viral infections, albinism, and possible mental health issues. Given the unique medical data that we are generating, we will conclude our data analyses by reviewing the medical findings and how they relate to witchcraft accusations, livelihood opportunities, chronic diseases, gender-disaggregated evidence(s), and our more memorable on-the-ground challenges.

Needless to say, as the locally obtuse *"Obroni,"* Richter and Flowers were quick to learn that we undeniably and repeatedly leaned on Dr. Salifu Bawa, Dr. Didier Amehi, Dr. Darko-Takyi, Gifty Mante, and many other local nurses and physicians to explain how we could most successfully distribute medications, ensure maximum comprehension, and enlist patient cooperation within the complex parameters of the multifaceted Ghanaian culture. As healthcare providers in N'gani, Richter and Flowers oftentimes needed two translators per American team member: One to translate from English to Konkomba, and another to translate from Konkomba to the more-obscure Dagomba language of Dagbani. Much like a medical version of the "telephone game"—where a single phrase is verbally passed along through a long line of people in order to laugh at how distorted the original message becomes after several people misquote and misunderstand the original phrase—

we never knew if our original query of "*How many times a day do you vomit?*" had mistakenly warped into a dialogue about menstruation, migraine headaches, or diarrhea! In our early years of medical outreach in Gnani, our patient-provider medical history and triage communications were (at best) a bit iffy in that our translators possessed very little medical terminology knowledge. Frustratingly, the majority of our rural Gnani patients appeared passively obedient (in an effort to appear polite, I suppose), repeatedly nodding in agreement, but we soon discovered that many patients had little understanding of the diagnosed disease or prescribed treatment(s) which usually included a wide array of colorful pills, sprays, lotions, and/or oral medications.

Without our knowledgeable local healthcare providers, we were ignorant to indigenous illnesses—especially in their nascent and "early" stages—unaccustomed to treating maladies like Buruli Ulcer, Guinea Worm, *kwashiorkor* (protein energy malnutrition or PEM), acute malnutrition, Leprosy (especially in their early stages), sky-high malarial fevers of 105° (usually accompanied by febrile seizures), and systolic blood pressures of 280 to 340 (which oftentimes exceeded the upper limits of our digital vital signs monitors, so we would attempt manual readings). The term *kwashiorkor* is from the Ghanaian Ga language meaning 'the sickness of the weaning' and usually strikes when a baby is weaned from protein-rich breast milk (as the subsequent baby must be breastfed) and switched to protein-poor foods (Geert 2007). In 1933 Cicely Williams was the first in Africa to describe *kwashiorkor*, a childhood nutritional disease concomitant of a low-protein, chiefly maize diet (Geert 2007). We witnessed many children with *kwashiorkor*, as they are easy to spot as their stomachs are bloated, their arms and legs are thin, their skin is flaky, and their hair loses its color (or has an orange-colored appearance). When you see these severely malnourished children, you immediately notice that they are dull-eyed, listless, slow, and devoid of energy to walk, run, or sometimes even lift up their head, legs, or arms, etc.

In fact, on the days we provided free medical care to the Konkomba people, our team members noted a much altered 'temperament' amongst the two ethnic groups, and for whatever reason(s) the Konkomba of Ghana are known as "one of Ghana's most fearsome northern people, often described as volatile, stubborn, and practically ungovernable" (Palmer 2010, 77). Ostensibly, among Ghanaian peoples, the Dagomba, Konkomba, and Mampurugu tribes are particularly engrossed and immersed in witchcraft beliefs (Npong 2014). Konkomba girls born into that community rarely receive a formal education, are "kept at home, doing all the household chores until their parents effectively sell them into servitude to another family through arranged marriage," and "most remain illiterate, vulnerable, and dependent for the rest of their lives" (Npong 2014, 1). These hostile opinions and lack of education and opportunities have surely augmented the general "paranoia,

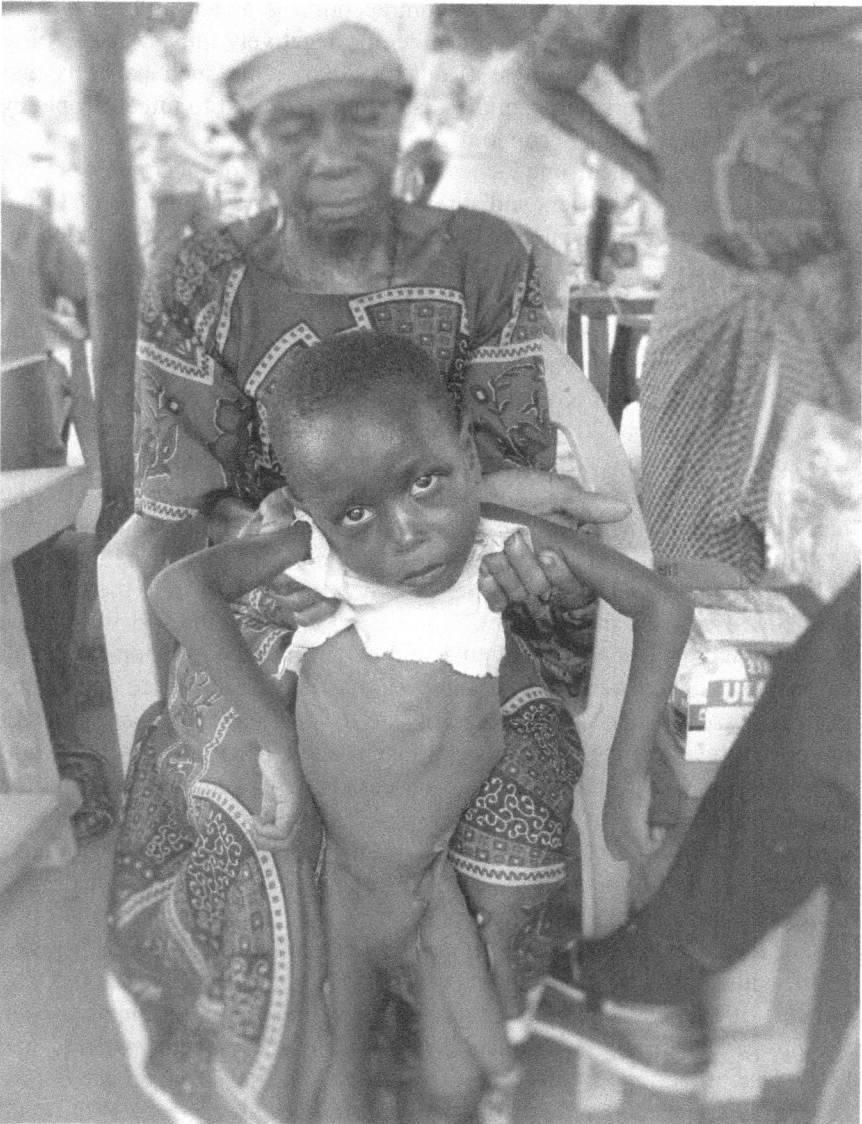

Figure 4.1. The long lines of women at a clinic for the Konkomba in Gnani in 2009.

isolation, and boredom that seems to blanket the north," and consequently, make these distant, socially removed, and isolated villages "ripe for accusations of witchcraft" (Palmer 2010, 77). Conspiracy theories also seem to abound in these remote regions concerning vaccinations and contraception; hidden plots and/or suspicions that contraception is a tool utilized by rich white people in order to sterilize or infect, or negatively impact, the fertility and/or growth of the powerless (Rodlach 2006). One such belief is that condom manufacturers purposefully distributed and used to infect people by adding lethal HIV germs to condoms.

In five large medical outreaches to Gnani—with (on average) approximately 8–12 clinical staffers and support persons—approximately 1,714 patients received free medical care. The breakout of patient numbers who received free medical and/or vision care is as follows: 194 patients were seen in late October through mid-November (after the rainy season) of 2007; 283 were treated in late October through mid-November of 2008; 245 in late October through mid-November of 2009; 437 in late October through mid-November of 2010 (262 Konkomba; 175 Dagomba; 60 de-wormed post clinic); and 555 in June of 2015. As a comprehensive example of how one annual outreach served patients breakdown: On the first day of our outreach, 157 Konkomba people were treated; on the second day, 207 were seen; on the third day 21 patients from the Gnani chief's family and entourage were treated; and on the fourth day 225 patients were treated in the Dagomba area including 5 in the vision clinic. The team then traveled down to the south to the Ekotsi-Bogyano area (where Richter is a Queen Mother) to work three consecutive days where 140 patients, 138 patients, and 40 (vision-only clinic) people received free medical and vision care, including free eye exams and eyeglasses. When deemed needed due to local (impure) water sources and/or outbreaks, at the end of (most) Gnani clinic tribal areas—the healthcare providers line up the remaining (unseen) patients and offer de-worming treatments—categorized of course by sex, age, and child-bearing age(s). Medical records are not kept of the people who are mass-treated with antiparasitics—but on average there are 300 locals that receive free de-worming medication donated by KINAPharma.

Our total number of patients from all five Gnani medical outreaches was 1,714; with adults (18 years old and older) constituting 1,022 (or about 59.62 percent) of the total number of patients. These numbers of patients broken out into gender-disaggregated data is 637 male (or 37 percent) patients, and 1,077 female (about 63 percent) patients. (See "Gender-Disaggregated Data for Gnani Patients 2007–2015" pie chart below.) The average age of the male patients (including children) was 24.85 years, and the average age of the female patients (including children) was 36.80 years. If we extrapolate the average age of adults (18 years old and older) only, the average age of the male adult patient was 52.76 years of age, and the average age of the adult female patient was 52.08 years of age. A further breakout of the adults seen at our clinics by age was as follows: ages 18–25 years (142 patients or 8.29

percent); ages 25–40 years (235 patients or about 13.72 percent); and age 40+ years (644 patients or about 37.57 percent).

In total, some 5,156 illnesses/trauma/diseases were clinically diagnosed by the WMP medical team throughout all the Gnani clinics (totaling 1,714 patients). One could hypothesize that the greater the number of illnesses/ traumas/diseases, the more ill (or in poor health) a patient was when they presented themselves at our triage. Conversely, the lower the number of complaints and/or illnesses treated, the healthier the resident. One significant factor—arguably the most critical factor—in the spread of disease is age, in that: "The older you get, the more susceptible you get. The very young and very old are the two major groups that are prone to infections" (Cochrane 2014, 1). Yet another significant factor, albeit nascent in its study, is gender-based differentials in health. Historically, only diseases related to women's reproductive and maternal functions have been studied, rather than sex- and gender-prevention(s) and treatment(s), which when proactively administered, could reduce women's excess health burdens and increase health equity. As Buvinić (et al) in *Disease Control Priorities in Developing Countries* argues:

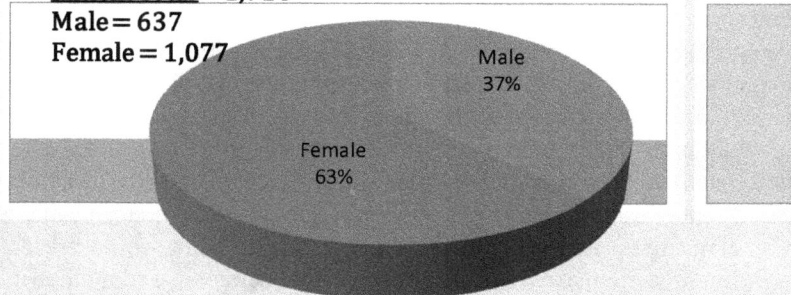

Figure 4.2. Gender-Disaggregated Data For Gnani Patients (2007–2015).

In health, more than in other social sectors, sex (biological) and gender (be-havioral and social) variables are acknowledged useful parameters for research and action because biological differences between the sexes determine male-specific and female-specific diseases and because behavioral differences be-tween the genders assign a critical role to women in relation to family health. (Buvinić et al. 2006)

In our clinics, the number of gender-disaggregated diagnoses among our 37 percent of male patients (adults at 286 and boys at 354) totaled 640, whereas among the 63 percent of female patients (adults at 696 and girls at 378) totaled 1,074. If we extrapolate the data further, we see that the adult women showed overall health inequities—as they presented with the highest number of treated illnesses, about three per woman (average age of 52, hence postmenopausal). We can also infer that male adults (with an average of 52 also) presented and were treated for an average of 2.66 illnesses/diseases, and male children and female children presented and were treated with 2.62 and 2.56 illnesses, respectively. As for standard deviations (σ—Greek sigma; the square root of the variance) of the 4 data sets (female adult, male adult, female pediatric, and male pediatric), adult women showed the highest standard deviation of 1.098. Of the four data sets, we found the following number of single diagnoses as: 27 among male adults, 60 for female adults, 41 for boys, and 51 for girls. For two diagnoses we reported 107 among male adults, 189 for female adults, 131 for boys, and 137 for girls. For patients reporting three diagnoses we reported 101 among male adults, 238 for female adults, 113 for boys, and 129 for girls. Patients who presented with four illnesses/diagnoses were: 39 among male adults, 150 for female adults, 59 for boys, and 52 for girls. Patients who were treated for five diagnoses were 12 among male adults, 54 for female adults, 10 for boys, and 8 for girls. Once again the female adult patients demonstrated a significant health inequity in that only females (5 adults and one child) were treated for the maximum of 6 illnesses. No male adult or male child presented and was recorded with 6 illnesses.

Accordingly, the number of diagnoses among adult females was 696, with a mean of 2.95, and a Standard Deviation (or measure of dispersion in a frequency distribution, equal to the square root of the mean of the squares of the deviations from the arithmetic mean of the distribution) of 1.098—our highest recorded deviation. Therefore, the average number of illnesses or treated diseases/traumas among the (average age 52) post-menopausal wom-en was about three illnesses. So the average female adult would present at triage with three diagnoses, such as hypertension, parasites, and malnutrition. (See "Female Adult Number of Diagnoses" next.)

In our clinics, the number of diagnoses among adult males was 286, with a mean of 2.66, and a Standard Deviation, or measure of the dispersion of

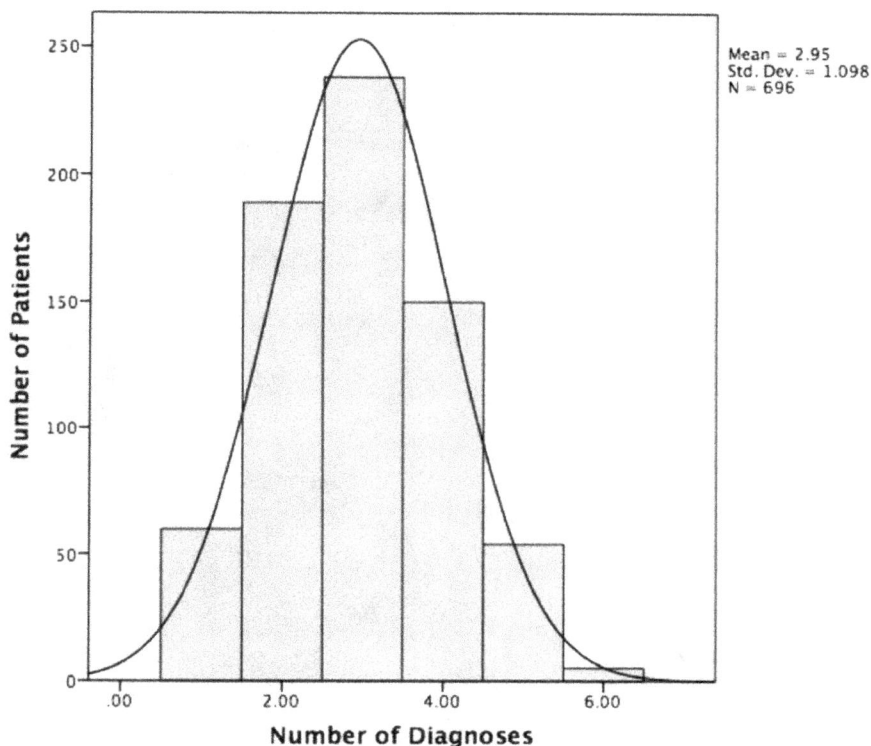

Figure 4.3. Female Adult Number of Diagnoses. Number of diagnoses 696; Mean = 2.95; with a Standard Deviation of 1.098.

this set of data from its mean, of .97. Therefore, the average number of illnesses or treated diseases/traumas among the men (average age 52.7—only slightly higher than our female average age of 52.0) was about 2 (or precisely 2.6) illnesses. As an example, the average male adult would present at triage with two diagnoses, such as back pain, and malaria. (See Chart 4.4 "Male Adult Number of Diagnoses" below.)

As for children (defined as patients under the age of 18 years), we treated 692 children (40.85 percent of patient total) with the following age distributions: ages under 2 years (208 patients or about 12.28 percent); ages 3–7 years (341 patients or about 20.13 percent); ages 8–12 years (102 patients or 6.02 percent); and ages 13–18 years (41 patients or about 2.42 percent). As for gender-disaggregated pediatric data, there were 378 girls (or 52 percent) and 354 boys (48 percent); indeed extremely equitable numbers of girl-to-

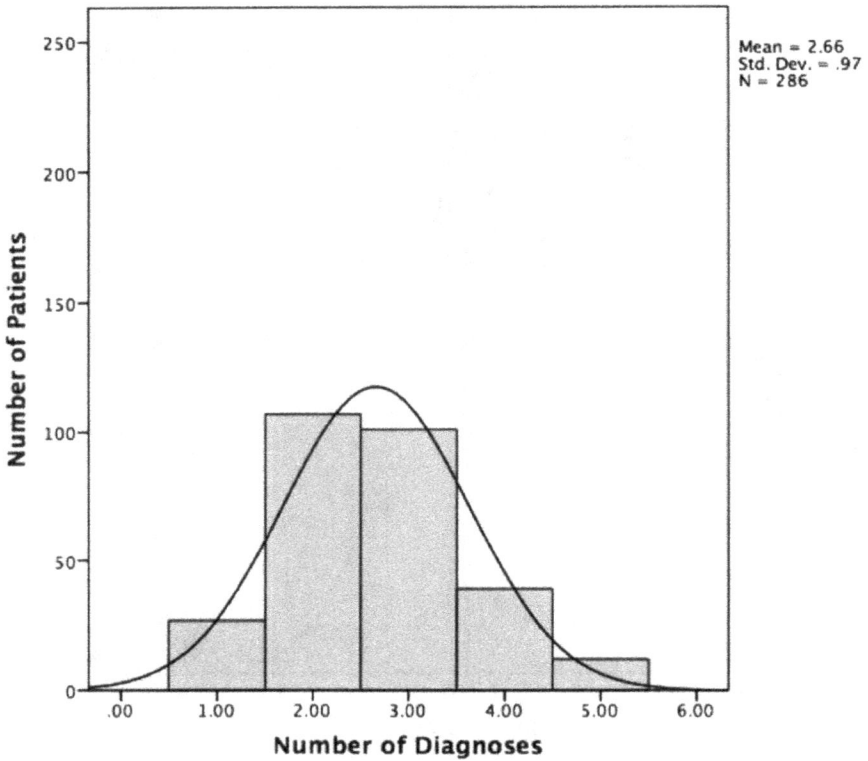

Figure 4.4. Male Adult Number of Diagnoses. Number of diagnoses 286; Mean = 2.66; with a Standard Deviation of .97.

boy ratios of patients. (See "Gender-Disaggregated Data for Pediatric Gnani Patients (Under the Age of 18) 2007–2015" in chart below.)

As for the range and number of treated illnesses/traumas (or diagnoses) among our 692 pediatric (under 18 years of age) patients: Young girls' and boys' diagnoses totaled 732, with 354 diagnoses among the boys, and 378 diagnoses among the girls. On average, young female girl patients exhibited 2.56 diagnoses, or illnesses/chief complaints that were treated. (See Chart 4.7 "Female Pediatric Number of Diagnoses.") Therefore, the average young female pediatric patient exhibited (on average) 2 to 3 diagnoses, or illnesses/chief complaints that were treated, such as malaria, parasites (gastrointestinal issues), and/or dehydration.

As for boys, our young male patients constituted 354 of our total diagnoses. On average, the boys at our clinics exhibited 2.62 (mean) diagnoses/illnesses/chief complaints that were treated, with a Standard Deviation of

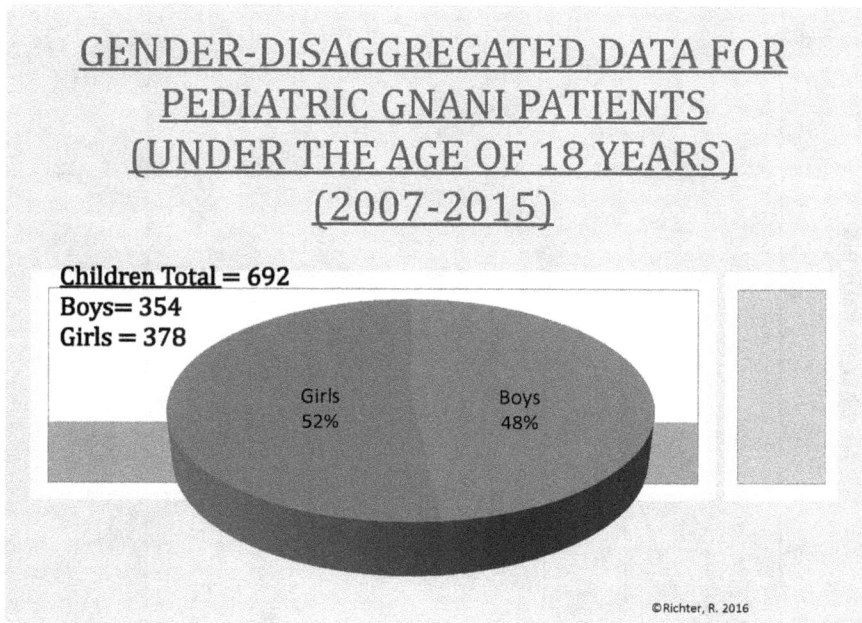

Figure 4.5. Gender-Disaggregated Data for Pediatric Gnani Patients (Under the Age of 18 Years).

.986. (See "Male Pediatric Number of Diagnoses.") Therefore, the average young male pediatric patient exhibited (on average) 2 to 3 diagnoses, or illnesses/chief complaints that were treated, such as malaria, conjunctivitis, and/or upper respiratory infection.

The types of ailments treated during our clinics varied by age and gender, but they inlcuded back pain and/or arthritis, gastrointestinal diseases like diarrhea, malaria, respiratory infections, bone and skin infections (especially from fieldworker-related trauma like ax/machete wounds on legs, arms, ankles, and/or feet), hypertension (which was extreme in many cases), and others. In general terms, these conditions can be broken down into trauma, and infectious and parasitic diseases, hypertension and cardiovascular disease, degenerative diseases, and diabetes. We also observed conditions such as epilepsy, mental health issues (i.e., depression, bipolar disorder, dementia, schizophrenia, anxiety disorders), and genetic syndromes (i.e., Down syndrome, autism, cystic fibrosis, albinism) that were the causes of people being condemned to the witches' villages. "In traditional communities there is no real understanding of depression or dementia," stated Dr. Akwesi Osei, chief

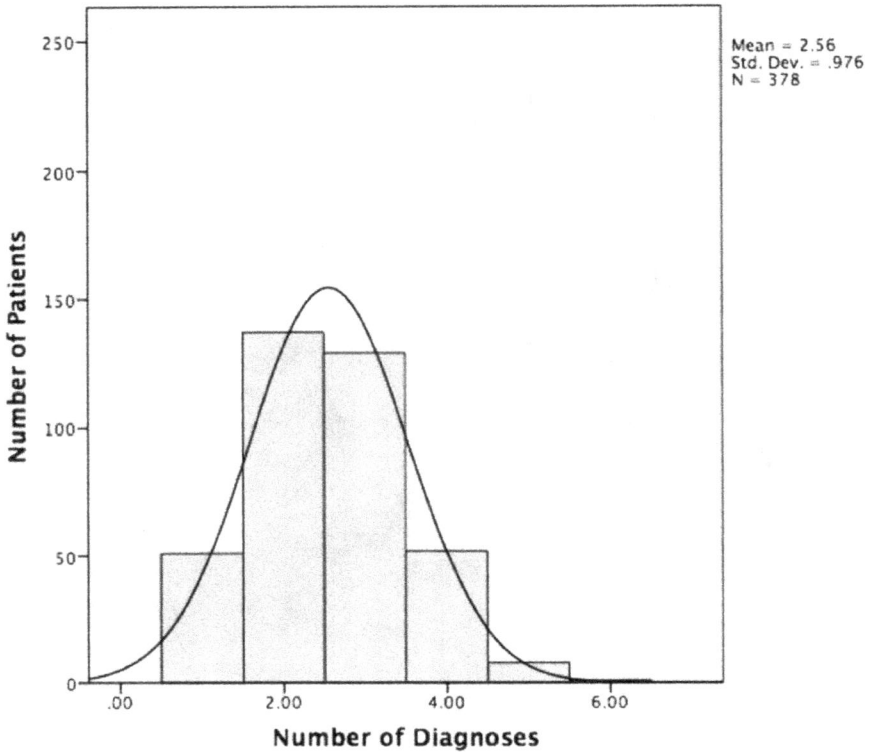

Figure 4.6.   Female Pediatric Number of Diagnoses. Number of diagnoses 378; Mean = 2.56; with a Standard Deviation of .976.

psychiatrist at the Ghana health service, who claims a majority of the women in the witches' camps have some sort of mental illness (Whitaker 2012, 1).

Abnormally high blood pressure, or hypertension, is usually defined as a repeatedly elevated blood pressure exceeding 140 mmHg over 90 mmHg (with a systolic pressure over 140 and/or or a diastolic pressure over 90 mmHg). However, for the purposes of this research we elevated our hypertension parameters to 145 mmHg (systolic) and/or 95 mmHg (diastolic) pressures. If either, or both, of the diastolic or systolic numbers were above the designated cut off numbers, they were included in our "extreme hypertensive" category. Out of 1,714 Gnani patients, 75 were recorded in this category. Some of the maximum recorded blood pressures in Gnani to date were primarily from older female residents: 233/135 mmHg, and 250/130 mmHg, and even a notable 254/145 mmHg. Oftentimes our battery-operated Propaq LT digital monitors would not register these extremely high pressures and we

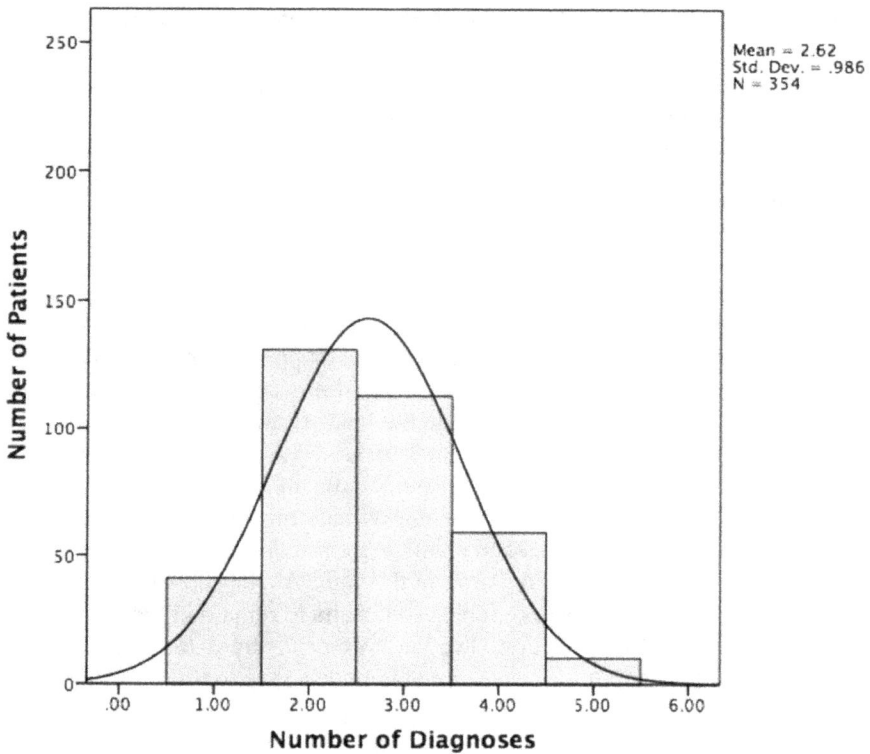

Figure 4.7. **Male Pediatric Number of Diagnoses. Number of diagnoses 354; Mean = 2.62; with a Standard Deviation of .986.**

were forced to take the blood pressures manually. According to many studies, chronic emotional and mental stress—such as anxiety, depression, and isolation from friends and family—are not only linked to heart disease, but are major cause(s) for hypertension as stress causes a sustained increase in the sympathetic nervous system that then accelerates pulse, contracts blood vessels, and increases blood pressure. As healthcare providers we can easily surmise that the extremely stressful living conditions in Gnani usher in record numbers of hypertensive cases since "the higher your psychological stress level, the higher your blood pressure is likely to be" (Mayo Clinic 2015, 1).

We must also recognize that our diagnoses, especially of infectious diseases were made on clinical presentation because in this very rural, undeveloped setting we were treating people in the shade of a tree with only the ability to take vital signs, and utilize a doppler, ultrasound, and check blood sugars via battery-operated equipment due to the lack of electricity, running water, room with walls, or even a microscope in these areas. We were aided in this endeavor by always having local physicians and nurses who were very familiar with endemic diseases. We also have the experience of working in the area multiple times as well as other remote regions in Africa such as Sierra Leone, Togo, South Africa, and Swaziland.

EXAMINATION OF GNANI PATIENT CONDITIONS

The compilation of this data occurred from short-term medical outreaches we performed as a part of the NGO World Missions Possible annually from 2007–2010 and again in 2015. We also had support from the Methodist Diocese of Northern Ghana and the Methodist minister from the local town of Yendi, providing us with meals for the team in the field, transportation, and other types of logistics such as translators.

Also we were only able to set up our clinics in the shade of a thatched roof, open air communal area at the one village and in the shade of three large trees at the other. Tables and chairs were provided by the villagers and we set up the "pharmacy" in and around the vans. As the sun would cross the sky, we would have to move our tables and chairs to remain in the shade.

To get to one of the locations, we had to cross a creek that was running across the road. The first year we were able to drive the van across because it was after the rainy season and nearly dried up but the following two years, the creek was too deep to drive the van across. The locals showed amazing adaptability as they carried motor bikes across and then we strapped boxes of equipment and medications on the front and back of the motor bikes which drove them the remaining three kilometers to the village. We crossed on a tree that had fallen across the stream and walked part of the way until the motor bikes, done ferrying the equipment, came back for us. Of course at the end of the day, this process had to be reversed.

All of our diagnoses were made clinically as we had no available diagnostics from a laboratory, CT scan, x-ray facilities, etc. Having African physicians and the nurse midwives were essential because of the different spectrum of illnesses that are seen in Ghana. In Gnani, we did have our own state-of-the-art vital sign monitors (monitoring pulse oximetry, EKG, temperatures, blood pressure, heart rate), as well as hospital-quality digital oral and tympanic thermometers, an automatic external defibrillator (AED), two handheld battery-operated obstetrical and vascular dopplers, otoscopes, stethoscopes, as well as digital autorefractors, focometers and ophthalmoscopes (panoptic and others) for vision diagnostics, and more. We have also utilized a 3.5 mHz ultrasound probe whose program was loaded onto our personal computer. However, we were immediately overrun with pregnant women seeking an ultrasound, and the unit could not keep up with the demand, and its battery quickly wore down–forcing the women to lay in the van's backseat while the doctors plugged the unit into the van's 12-volt cigarette lighter for power. Dr. Flowers remembers telling one woman that she was pregnant with twins, and the woman's response was subdued distress. Either her concern was having two, not one, more mouth to feed, or facing the taboo of multiple births in the northern region. (See in-depth discussion of "The Curse of Multiple Births.")

Soil-transmitted Helminths are very common in sub-Saharan Africa (WACIPAC 2003). These parasitic infections are caused by poor sanitation and exposure through ingesting food or water contaminated with fecal material. In some cases such as hookworms, the spores can enter through skin exposed to contaminated soil. The people in Gnani live in a 'textbook environment' rife with these particular parasitic infections. The treatment of these worms usually involves a single dose of anti-parasitic medication, such as Mebendazole or Albendazole. It was the consensus of our indigenous and American medical team members that we would take the opportunity to administer anti-helminthic treatment to any patient for whom the treatment was not contraindicated. Hence the reason that the most common type of medication prescribed by our team were anti-helminthic drugs. This approach has been widely used by other organizations such as the WHO, the FRESH program of the World Bank, and UNICEF (focused on school-age children) (WACIPC 2003). The hindrance in these programs is that it can be slow to reach and/or penetrate rural, hard-to-reach areas such as Gnani. We were generously given these medications in great quantity by Kina Pharma, LTD of Ghana. We treated 1,056 (recorded) patients with anti-helminthic medication. Sometimes there were contraindications such as pregnancy, age, hypersensitivity, drug interactions, multiple medication intolerance(s), or other condition(s). (See "Diagnoses / Conditions Treated 2007–2015" chart.) The next most common condition treated was fever (758 patients, 44.2 percent). We considered a fever to be 99.1 or above. Many times the fever was treated as a part of the treatment for malaria, respiratory infections, gastroenteritis, etc. The drugs we used for treatment of fever were acetaminophen or ibuprofen based on the age of the patient. There were a few children who presented with febrile seizures all of whom were successfully treated with fever control.

The third most common disease which we treated was malaria (614 patients, 35.6 percent), again diagnosed clinically due to the lack of diagnostic capability. This is in alignment with published data showing malaria to be a major public health problem in Ghana. The country as well as neighboring countries has been battling this problem for decades. Serious attempts to control malaria began in Ghana in the 1950s, according to the Ghana Health Service (2009). Interventions enacted during this time included insecticides, mass chemoprophylaxis and improvements in the drainage system. Despite these measures malaria has remained the leading cause of illness in the country. (For more information on malaria, see "Common Disease of Malaria.")

The patients presented with fever, sweats, headache, and "waist pain" which we would consider back pain or myalgias. Sometimes they would have nausea and vomiting. Again, Kina Pharma LTD provided an abundance of medication for both adults and children for malaria. If a patient is pregnant, they are supposed to take intermittent preventive treatment (IPT) at least twice during the pregnancy. Therefore, we could provide this medication for our pregnant patients.

Our next highest category of treatment was acute gastroenteritis (429 patients, 25 percent). This is to be expected given the extreme poverty in which these people live, the poor hygiene, and the improper disposal of human waste (which invariably leads to a contamination of the water supply).

A significant number of patients, 270 or 66 percent, were sick enough to require specific treatment for dehydration using anti-nausea medication and rehydration solution. We use large quantities of a particular rice-based, gluten-free oral electrolyte solution (ORS) containing varying levels of sodium and carbohydrates for adults and pediatric patients (CeraLyte 50/70/90). We only use these ORS solutions that utilize mixed-chain carbohydrates (maximize rapid absorption; maintain low osmolarity) to provide the right absorptions of electrolytes to these patients—therefore decreasing our need for field IV rehydration therapy (where IVs are impractical and present unsterile conditions). Gnani residents fetch their water from a nearby river, and do not have effective sterilization methods, so they are constantly being exposed to water-borne illnesses such as Salmonella. In 2015, this was a particularly prominent problem among the Dagomba as there had been some recent flooding and the vast majority of the children were ill with diarrheal illnesses. Most of our patients treated with oral rehydration therapy (270 patients or 15.7 percent) were also gastroenteritis patients who required this particular treatment for immediate rehydration.

We treated 357 (approximately 20.8 percent) patients for respiratory infections. Our medical team members always take precautions to wear N-95 masks (resistant to Tuberculosis). Recent data indicates that the prevalence of TB is much higher than previously estimated. In 2014 a study showed that there were 286 cases per 100,000 people in Ghana, with prior estimates by the WHO at 92 cases per 100,000 people, according to the Ghana News Agency (2015). The mortality is 7.5 per 1,000 infected, and the news agency reported that 2014 surveyed increase in prevalence was due to the synergistic relationship with HIV/AIDS (2015). As we were without laboratory testing for tuberculosis or HIV/AIDS, we treated based upon clinical diagnoses. A

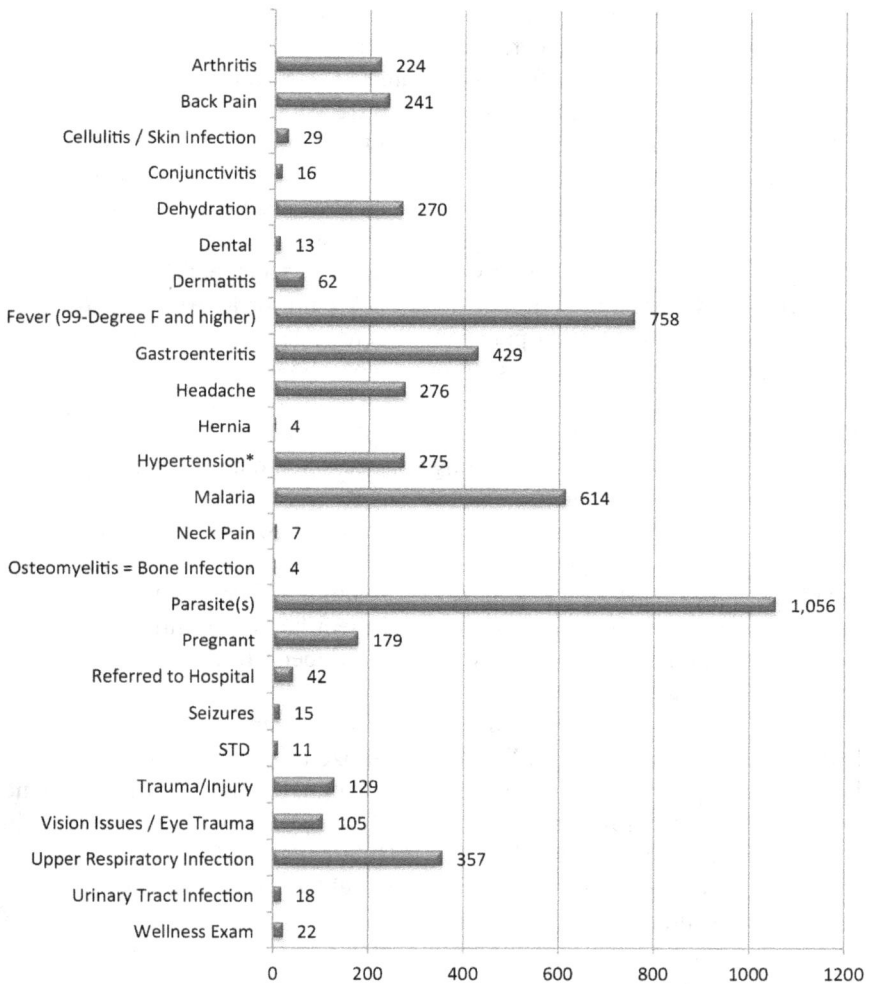

Figure 4.8. Diagnoses/Conditions Treated 2007–2015.

few of these patients were coughing up blood, so our suspicion for TB was high, and they were immediately referred to the local hospitals with TB programs (such as Yendi Hospital) for treatment. In most acute referral cases, WMP would pay for the patient's transport, and/or enrollment into the national healthcare insurance scheme, and/or hospital care, depending on the patient's diagnosis and expected prognosis.

There were 276 patients (approximately 16.1 percent) treated for headaches. Frequently the headache was due to the symptoms of another illness such as malaria, fever, or respiratory infection, etc. In none of our cases was there a sudden onset of a severe headache or symptomatology or findings suggestive of a neurologic emergency (such as intracranial bleeding, etc.).

Hypertension was identified and treated in 275 (approximately 16 percent) of the patients. Some of these values were astonishingly high, e.g., 275/150. Very few of these hypertensive patients were aware of their hypertension and under medical treatment. This was yet another telling example of the toll that the lack of access to proper medical care is taking on these Gnani residents. There were some 5–10 patients who were partially paralyzed, living with the sequelae from a prior Cerebrovascular accident (CVA).

A relatively common complaint was back pain, or as we were to learn, their terminology was "waist pain." We treated 241 patients (approximately 14 percent) for back pain. It was a rare patient who had any history of injury and no one who seemed to have any serious problem such as radiculopathy. This seemed to be the favored "chief complaint" of the few healthy young men in their 20s who were attempting to access some complimentary medication and/or gratis treatment.

Arthritis was a chief complaint among these predominantly elderly women. Over 224 patients (approximately 13 percent of the total) who presented themselves were treated for arthritic complaints. Of course these arthritic patients tended to be elderly, and some of them had deformities from prior (untreated) limb fractures and injuries that improperly healed due to a lack of proper medical treatment.

Of the women, only 179 (approximately 25 percent of the adult women) had self-reported as pregnant. We did not utilize urine pregnancy test kits as it would have proven unmanageable to have women urinate (as there were no "restrooms" anywhere), and then (somehow) have them resume their place in line so we could read the results of an early pregnancy. When you consider that majority of the women we treated were elderly and well beyond childbearing years, the remaining percentage of women in the child-bearing age group was very high. We were able to check fetal heart tones with one of our two battery-operated Doppler Fetal Monitors. Most of the pregnant women in Gnani were awestruck and excited to hear their baby's fetal heart tones for the first time.

Trauma and injuries accounted for 129 patients (approximately 7 percent of Gnani patient total) in our clinics. Most of these patients presented with fractures that had healed improperly—but the injuries were usually more than 6 months old, so we could do no more than treat for residual pain. There were several occasions where medical team members were close to vomiting from the overwhelming stench of open wounds that were wrapped with any variety of "herbal cures" that were usually composed of compacted mud, unsterile grasses, herbs, and necrotizing flesh (dead tissue, and wound debris). The "traditional cures" we witnessed usually contained mud, which could contaminate the wound with fragments of human waste, bacteria, organic foreign bodies, irritants, and contribute to wound infection. These traditional poultices run in direct opposition to Western wound care practices, which dictate that wounds should be kept clean, devoid of plant matter, and dirt, and irrigation of an open wound is the preferred method in evidence-based medicine in modern wound care (Bauman 2007). Although it should be noted that *some* clays have been found hold antibacterial properties capable of killing pathogens (like E. coli, and methicillin-resistant Staphylococcus aureus, a.k.a., MRSA), yet (untested) clay use can also topically introduce very dangerous lead, mercury, and arsenic into a patient's bloodstream (Otto and Haydel 2013).

Vision issues were diagnosed in 105 (approximately 6 percent) of our clinic patients. These consisted of primarily cataracts, retinal detachments, river blindness, trachoma, and other visual impairment issues. One unforgettably disheartening case was a young 26 year-old Ghanaian woman we saw in Ekotsi-Bogyano had been permanently blinded in both eyes in a domestic violence assault. It was not uncommon for women—young and old—to present themselves at our clinics with (one or two) retinal detachments, torn retinas, or retinal hemorrhages after being violently shaken (known as "adult shaken syndrome"; forceful head jerking), falling from 50 feet or more, or being violently struck in the face, eye(s), or head by her husband or significant other.

There were 62 patients (3.6 percent) who were treated for various types of dermatitis. We also had 29 cases of cellulitis and about four cases of osteomyelitis (bone infections) with chronic open wounds. Additionally, there were 18 patients, mostly women with symptoms of urinary tract infection. We treated 16 patients, mostly children for conjunctivitis, and 13 patients for toothache. Fifteen patients had a history of epilepsy although only one had a seizure at the clinic. Eleven patients were treated for Sexually Transmitted Disease. Most of these were men with the complaint of penile discharge, so we treated them with conventional antibiotics against gonorrhea and chlamydial infections. We also advised that they inform their sex partner—about 1/3 of the men brought their wives or girlfriends in for treatment.

Some seven patients were treated for "neck pain," although none had a history of recent injury. There were also four patients identified with hernias, which we referred to the hospital for surgical intervention. In total, there were approximately 42 patients referred to local hospitals, usually Yendi Hospital. Many of them were for treatment of their hypertension, and four (as mentioned above) were sent for hernia surgery evaluations. One of these patients was acutely ill and she was transported to a hospital for hypovolemic shock due to infection or gastroenteritis.

Here it should also be noted that 1,041 patients also received some form of vitamins. We dispensed primarily KinaPharma's adult "Fine Life" Blood

Tonic, "Fine Life" B Complex, Mayfer prenatal syrup, pediatric multi-vitamin syrup, and adult multi-vitamin syrups. Unless contraindicated, every patient received some form of a multi-vitamin supplement in an attempt to decrease local cases of: anemia, weak bone, muscle, and nerve function (due to calcium deficiencies); rickets (caused by vitamin D deficiencies); birth defects (caused by folate/folic acid deficiencies during pregnancy), and many other illnesses and malformations caused by a nutrient-poor diet.

While we didn't have the resources and/or manpower to perform immunizations, the Ghanaian government has active immunization program(s) and there are many community health workers who do perform these function(s) and more even in the remote area of Gnani. In 2008, the local nurse and community health workers heard about our huge turn-out and asked if we would be willing to allow them to "piggy-back" their services with our clinic. Of course we wholeheartedly agreed and they performed immunizations while people waited in our clinic lines. It was an exceptional 100 percent win-win scenario for both the patients and the healthcare providers.

We're familiar with the fact that these people, who are among the poorest of the poor, often ingest contaminated water without boiling it or sterilizing it in any way and are frequently infected with water-borne parasites. The common parasites in Ghana include (but are not limited to) the following: water-contact disease of schistosomiasis; Typhoid and Cholera via consumed contaminated food and water; the intestinal parasite *Giardia lamblia*; Onchocerciasis (a.k.a., "river blindness" caused by the parasitic worm *Onchocerca volvulus*), hookworms, roundworms (like lymphatic Filariasis), and numerous others. There is a medically significant and long-reported association between malnutrition and parasitic infections. Consequently when considering the evaluation for the widespread administration of anti-helminthic drugs to persons residing in remote sub-Saharan areas, there is an abundance of literature to show that these parasitic infections are very widespread and exacerbate the residents' pre-existing poor nutrition–all contributing to a vicious intergenerational succession of growth failure via anemia, wasting/stunting of growth, low-birth-weight/intrauterine growth retardation, and a 'failure to thrive.' It is also common for children to be infected by more than one type of worm (Papier et al. 2014). The reasons for the worsening of malnutrition due to parasitic infections include anorexia, and nutrient wastage through blood loss, diarrhea, and/or vomiting (Lwanga et al. 2012). We did come prepared to provide anti-parasitic medication to everyone who presented themselves to our clinics, unless of course, it was contraindicated (i.e., pregnancy, age, hypersensitivity, etc.). For instance, on our most recent trip, in June of 2015, one of the villages we visited had an outbreak of diarrhea from drinking the contaminated river water. Nearly everyone was suffering from diarrhea. Our Ghanaian nurse Gifty Mante provided a teaching session to the women at the clinic, telling them that the river water was making them sick and how to sterilize the water. Interestingly, we spoke to representative of another NGO that provided "clay-pot filters" which are very simple to use and made in Ghana. We know that in some communities, people refuse to drink pre-boiled or filtered water because they explained to us that it "tastes bad." One of the precautions we had to make was to be sure to take lots of bottled water to use for mixing children's antibiotics, rehydration salts, etc. There were many fights among the residents and children over the empty water bottles.

We are grateful to have enjoyed a remarkable relationship with Kofi Nsiah Poku, CEO of Kina Pharma, a wholly Ghanaian owned and operated pharmaceutical manufacturing distribution and marketing company in Accra, Ghana. Every year Poku and Kina Pharma donates a truckload of various medications such as anti-parasitic (anti-Malarial), antibiotic medications, gastrointestinal medicines, multivitamins, prenatal vitamins, nonsteroidal anti-inflammatory drugs (NSAID), and other non-narcotic medications. Wherever our World Missions Possible team worked, team doctors were able to donate excess medication(s) for use at local public hospitals and non-private clinics.

On-the-Ground Medical Challenges and Lessons Learned

Needless to say, as American Obroni, we made some enormous (and in retrospect somewhat amusing) cultural missteps and miscalculations along the way. Indeed, there are far too many that come to mind, so we will only briefly mention some of the most multi-culturally indicative and didactic accounts. They also illustrate that no matter how much you painstakingly organize and prepare your international medical teams, there are always surprises. As Richter, president of World Missions Possible stated: "What's most needed in international field work is a selfless motivation paired with endless flexibility. That makes not only the medical fieldworker effective, but also keeps the rest of the team happy." Since 2001, World Missions Possible has provided aid, vision care, and EMS training/capacity building in hard-to-reach, overlooked, and underserved rural areas in 16 developing nations (including Bulgaria, Burundi, Costa Rica, El Salvador, Ghana, India, Nicaragua, Mexico, Sierra Leone, South Africa, Swaziland, Togo, Uganda, USA, Vietnam, and Zambia). To date, WMP has provided approximately 590 surgeries, 5,560 medical exams and care, 6,000 eye exams, and distributed over 7,750 free pairs of eyeglasses—all free of charge to the patients. The organization, which averages 3 percent to 5 percent administrative costs, has been recognized as "Best in America" by Independent Charities of America, and is a proud member of U.S.A.'s Combined Federal Campaign "Charities Under 5 percent Overhead."

On WMP's first medical outreach to Ghana in 2006, we arranged for a local Ghanaian in Houston to laboriously translate medication and patient discharge instructions in Twi, Ghana's most widely spoken language. For weeks thereafter, we brainstormed and came up with 15 or 20 diagnoses that we expected to encounter (malaria, diarrhea, fever, dehydration, etc.) and then developed treatment and "take-home" medication handouts. We then racked our brains deciding on "how-to" diagrams: Pills versus tablets; sun versus moon; and bloody diarrhea versus bloody urine pictograms. With a self-satisfaction that originates in naiveté, we then traveled with hundreds of copies, all dutifully alphabetized into a single enormous 50-tab file folder, to Ghana. But when we drove 16 hours out into the remote Northern Region villages, we discovered that there are somewhere around 250 languages and dialects in Ghana, and the vast majority of our patients didn't speak English, or Twi, and countless more were either illiterate or semi-literate. So much for our 'innovative' take-home medication instructions! They were, in fact, terribly impractical and disastrously ineffectual.

Yet another universal challenge for us, wherever we go, are the very long lines of patients waiting to be seen. Many of our Ghanaian patients in these remote villages had never seen a medical doctor—and some of them had never met a white person, so children are known to shout "fada" (father) as their primary exposure to white people has been a religious pastor, or "father." Richter's blonde hair (locally referred to as "spider webs") always proves to be quite a novelty, so she always wears a hat to minimize attention to her hair. We also consistently encounter problems with the crowds encroaching on us. At one of our "Clinic Without Walls" (as we refer to them) in Lawra (Upper West Region of Ghana, bordering Burkina Faso), the crowds became so desperate to reach the clinic that two men were forced to beat back the crowds away from the medical team with palm fronds so they could perform their tasks needed to conduct the clinic. Sometimes the medical team sets up under the shade of a tree; other times under a thatched roof (without walls), or in an open-air building. In Gnani, the women bring these tiny little footstools to sit on and continuously edge closer and closer, crowding and surrounding the healthcare providers. There is a lot of shouting, arguing, and generalized chatter from the crowds—usually making the din tremendous. Luckily our medical team has state-of-the-art, battery-powered electronic vital signs monitors as it would prove impossible to triage the volume of patients we see if we had to manually auscultate patients' blood pressures.

In order to be assured of care, some of the women would feign a faint—only to jump up with excitement when we began to approach them. But we soon became savvy to the diversions. For those patients who were waiting in line—for the novel experience, sheer boredom, or hope of "free stuff" from the American *Obroni* doctors, we provide vitamins, toothbrushes, and anti-

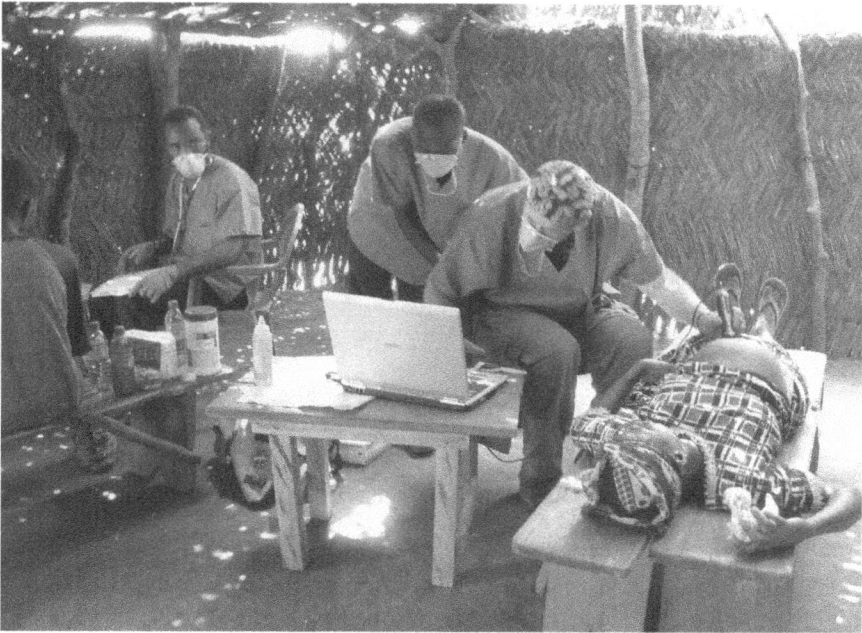

Figure 4.9.   In 2008, Dr. Flowers using a high-tech PC-powered ultrasound in a goat hut.

parasitic medicine. This gives us the opportunity to provide useful wellness and hygiene "freebies" to these patients. It was, unfortunately, very commonplace for patients to request "medicine" for a family member or neighbor who was not present at the clinic.

We were constantly having to hire and pay translators to be able to ask questions of the patients as well as give them information and instructions. Frequently children would be brought by people who were unrelated and didn't know anything about the child's chief complaint or medical history. It was always challenging to get the history because frequently they wouldn't know it and we had to ask questions sometimes through two translators.

Before our first Gnani outreach, we effected months of brainstorming. As healthcare providers, our principal concern was to adhere to the First Rule of Medicine: "Do No Harm." As an example, it is well documented that if you start a patient on a blood-pressure medicine (and they discontinue or run out of them), it is possible to have a severe rebound effect, increasing the person's blood pressure, potentially precipitating a complication such as a heart attack or stroke. In this case, you could unintentionally cause one of the problems you were, in fact, attempting to prevent. From our very first out-

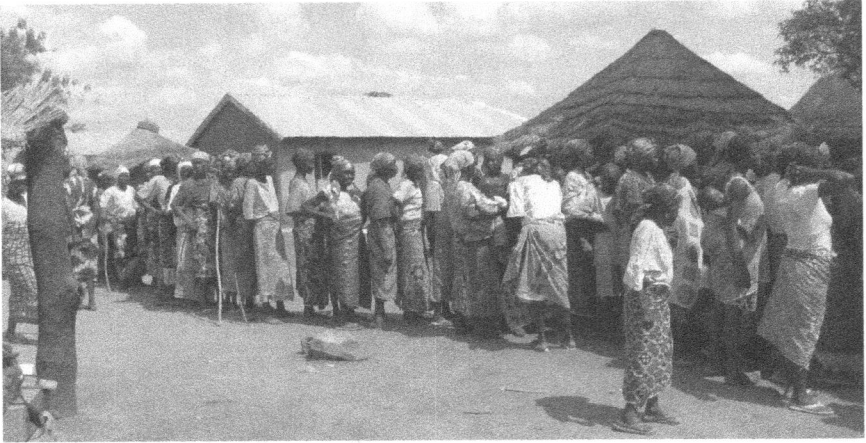

Figure 4.10. Long lines of Konkomba women waiting in line for free medical care in Gnani.

reach, we made the decision to only notify patients of their hypertension—and then donate the necessary drugs to a nearby clinic or hospital (such as Yendi Hospital) so they could receive appropriate follow-up care, conscientious treatment, and free medication. We would instruct hospital administrators that any of the patients we sent in for long-term treatment should receive our (donated medication) without cost, and they could utilize the balance of cases of donated medications.

We have been fortunate that we had the support of KinaPharma, a Ghana-based pharmaceutical manufacturer who provided donated medicines by the truckload—from antibiotics and anti-malarials to non-narcotic pain medicines, stomach medicines, etc. However, we were very concerned that the patients who might be needing treatment for pain (with acetaminophen or an anti-inflammatory medicine) might take a potentially toxic dose. And certainly, this was a predominant concern for all of the medicines we dispensed, so our team only dispensed less-than-toxic/non-toxic amounts of medications—so if the patient were to (erroneously) ingest the entire content, they would remain unharmed. Certain donated medications were donated to clinics and hospitals so that they would be administered by attending clinical care professionals.

One type of medicine that we used was rectal suppositories for children (acetaminophen for fever, and Tigan, an anti-nausea medication). During our clinics, we would often encounter young babies and children in the midst of febrile (Malarial) seizures; vomiting and unable to digest oral medicines. The febrile seizures in this rural fieldwork were alarming, as we could only "cool" them down with our small supplies of tepid bottled water and administer medications. One problem we had not anticipated (due to the immense heat and shirt-drenching humidity) was that these rectal suppositories would crumble into multiple pieces when we pried opened the blister packs. So sometimes we had 4–6 slippery pieces of a single suppository dose to rectally insert into a struggling and screaming infant. After our clinics, Flowers and Richter would occasionally commiserate and giggle about what these isolated villagers thought about our "high-tech American medicine," which included inserting medicine (multiple times) into their baby's rectum!

We also made sure that whenever we were treating with pediatric oral antibiotics or oral rehydration solution (ORS), which come in bottles and packets and must be reconstituted, that we mixed the medications with bottled water and had them drink the contents in the presence of our Ghanaian nurse. It would be illogical to prescribe medications to counteract gastrointestinal parasites or illnesses due to contaminated water by using contaminated water! For pediatric solutions, we would dispense a 5 ml. syringe and mark the child's specified dose in black indelible ink. We also began to dispense individual bags (one for each patient), as was often the case that each grandmother or mother would bring two or three children for us to treat. The dispensing nurse would have to explain that the medication was not to be shared with other "sick" family members or sold to others who were ill as the medication was specifically for them and would not work for anyone else.

Perhaps one of the most memorable moments occurred after the Wenchi area held a *"semi-Durbar"* for Flowers and Richter for the donation of an EKG and Automatic External Defibrillator (AED) and other resuscitation/EMS materials to the Wenchi Methodist (public) Hospital in the Brong-Ahafo Region in Ghana. (A Ghanaian *Durbar* is a traditional festival where chiefs and other prominent officials are present—ours in Wenchi was a smaller tented affair with local chiefs, local hospital officials, media, etc.) After the semi-*Durbar*, WMP offered several sessions teaching resuscitation techniques to hospital staff in: CPR (with an American Red Cross nurse from USA); and EKG Interpretation on the WMP-donated EKG. Dr. Richter, as a Ghanaian Queen Mother, was asked to travel out to meet with local officials and dignitaries to be formally welcomed. Richter arrived to a roomful of regional elders. The traditional leader was in his late 80s and blind. He asked the translator what Richter looked like, and the roomful of elders chuckled when the leaders explained that Richter resembled a "young Julie Andrews." Richter was then asked to speak about WMP, its work, and then finally, to explain (in layman's terms) what this brand-new, high-tech donated medical equipment did. Richter knew she needed to choose her words carefully in describing a machine that could potentially 'fix' a heart that had stopped beating. After a lengthy explanation (with many hedged statements), the room was quiet, thoughtful, and then filled with excited whispers. When

Richter asked the translators what the local officials understood of the state-of-the technology, they said that the chiefs were thrilled to have a real-life "resurrection machine" in their city. To little avail, Richter spent the rest of the session attempting to tame the crowd's enthusiasm, potential life-saving capabilities, and lofty expectations of their new AED. Later, one of the local doctors told Richter that the locals "will be bringing in dead people for months." Which, in fact, was the actual case—until locals and officials began to understand much more about their celebrated "resurrection machine."

One of our most troublesome issues, year after year, was how to safely manage and (to a certain extent) carry out triage for the most ill. Triage, or the assessment and assignment of care in a prioritized order of treatment, remained absolutely unmanageable. Everyone expected their coveted "next" place in line to be respected—with zero tolerance allotted for others in line needing more urgent medical care. In 2008, we tried to quell arguments in line by creating a "numbered system" where each patient received a slip of paper with numbers from 1 to 50, re-using those numbers as the patients were seen. The next day we chuckled a lot when many new patients stood in line with their own homemade slips of paper, stating numbers between 2 and 700! So, in (yet another) effort to move our more acute cases (the handicapped, very old, and/or extremely weak) to the front of our lines, Richter adopted her aptly named "sneaky triage" system in 2009. The open, public assign-ment of triage (a prioritized order of treatment based on degrees of urgency for care—was unmistakably impossible in these (already) hyper-chaotic set-tings. The essence of Richter's "sneaky triage" is simple: Have all medical team members walk through the lines of people, greeting them with hand-clapping and a native-tongue "hello"—while noting any corporeal signs of illness and/or trauma such as: rashes, ringworm, malnutrition ("orange" hair, bloated bellies, etc.), listlessness (especially in babies and/or children), high fever (checked with back of wrist), inability to walk or stand, obvious trau-ma, eye redness, and more. On the "second round" of greeting, these observ-ably ill patients obtain wipe-off trauma tags which are clipped onto their clothing. If the crowds are especially chaotic, terms such as "60 y/o F—R leg INF" are written on tag so the tags cannot be switched and/or re-used by others (notation for an elderly woman who has infection on right leg). At various times (and discreetly) during the clinic, these "pre-screened" patients are helped to the triage waiting area, ensuring that they will receive care that day. This flawed and imperfect system allows the medical team to locate some of the more obviously (albeit physically evident) ill patients—that typically get pushed to the back of the line as they are the weakest, most disabled, and acutely ill of all of the people waiting in line.

Of course, our cultural missteps were (and are) too numerous to individu-ally mention. Some experiences we considered heartbreaking and others we considered profound teaching moments where we were akin to coal—tested, heated, and hard-pressed into diamonds—in the hot and arduous "fires" of humanitarian fieldwork.

Chapter Five

Pathologies of Prejudice in Social Mechanisms

Gender-based violence in Ghana gags its elderly widows, assertive business-women, liberated feminists, and childless brides like an antiquated muzzle: Inciting fear, silencing public outcry, and eliciting manifest submission. It is an enduring stranglehold composed of intermingled fiscal, gender, cultural, religious, patriarchal, and social tourniquets. And much like the glow-in-the-dark orange grease that stains your plate from the ubiquitous carrot-colored Ghanaian palm nut oil—gendered violence permeates and tarnishes the country's global standing, human rights record, social fabric, and national economy.

As healthcare providers, social scientists, and humanitarian aid laborers, we possess a moral and professional obligation to tell these stories of our sisters in social bondage. It is patently obvious to anyone (with or without the sparsest of medical knowledge basics) that these aged women are sickly, malnourished, depressed, anemic, fatigued, destitute, and without hope. They also suffer from acute hypertension from the stressful environ, poor vision and blindness from untreated cataracts, crippling osteoarthritis, and other illnesses that typically befall any elderly person who works hard physical labor with insufficient access to nourishing food, or medical, dental, or eye care. Most are involved in polygamous marriages; receive little to no financial support, access to prudent legal advice, civil remedies, or any jurisdictional redress. Therefore in curious retrospect: Is it any wonder that poor, uneducated, disrespected, defenseless, economically disenfranchised, and socially/fiscally/politically powerless women with little self-esteem have relished (and even welcomed) the absolute respect, untamed fear, and limitless power that belongs to the mystery of witchcraft?

According to the U.S. Department of State, some of the most important human rights problems in Ghana in 2014 included "violence against women and children including female genital mutilation/cutting," and "societal discrimination against women" (2014, 1).

According to Ter Haar's estimates of the inhabitants, the "majority of them are women," and the Commission for Human Rights and Administrative Justice (CHRAJ) noted in 1998 that out of 815 condemned people in Ghanaian witches' villages, only 13 were male (Ter Haar 2007, 72). Therefore in this chapter we will explore the ways gender-based violence and structural violence against women adversely affects human rights, equitable educational opportunities, healthcare access and outcomes, social authority, political rights, the nation's aged population, and the Ghanaian economy.

Conversely, it should be noted that in some societies men can find themselves—in an atypical role reversal—as the predominantly accused gender. Researchers such as Diane Ciekawy (1999) and Rosalind Shaw (1985) have shown the men in the Mijikenda in Kenya and the Temne women in Sierra Leone are both proactive agents in the condemnation of men and in the divination consultations involved in witchcraft accusations, respectively (Damasane 2009).

STRUCTURAL VIOLENCE

Mahatma Gandhi famously referred to poverty as "the worst form of violence," however violence can be manifested in a host of forms of direct (obvious, sporadic, carried out by identifiable individual[s] for intentional harm), domestic, structural (avoidable, not always obvious, almost always invisible, can be unintentional, and carried out continuously by systematic social, political, or economic efforts, and/or embedded in institutions), and cultural—with structural violence existing as the more obscure, opaque, and indistinct form of manifested violence, oftentimes cloaked in ubiquitous practices whereby the harm is more protracted, indirect, commonplace, problematic to comprehend in scope, and provide any reparation for damages (Richter 2015). Richter goes on to note that structural violence ensues when people are "affected, injured, or impaired due to inequitable social composition" (as opposed to direct physical violence), and this systemic violence "occurs when an institutionalized practice, scheme, or established system negatively impacts groups in an inequitable fashion, whereby people are socially, politically, and/or economically exploited, oppressed, and dominated" (Richter 2015). A few examples of structural violence include: elitism, ethnocentrism, classism, racism, sexism, nationalism, heterosexism, and ageism, or any other form of exploitation, poverty, denial of basic needs, or marginalization of a person(s) in witches' villages. Johan Galtung first coined the term "structural violence" in the 1960s and explained that "unequal life chances" usher in inequitable accesses to resources, political power, education, healthcare, or legal status. "I understand violence as the avoidable impairment of fundamental human needs," and the "impairment of human life, which lowers the actual degree to which someone is able to meet their needs below that which would otherwise be possible" (Galtung 1993, 106).

Consequently, structural violence—in all of its forms—fabricates pronounced and preventable causes of premature death, suffering, needless disabilities, as well as the exacerbation of lower acuity illnesses/diseases into higher acuity illness/disease phases (Richter 2015). As we see from this research, the condemned witches fall victim to structural violence in that their access to life-saving emergency medical care is obstructed, discouraged, and/or flatly denied by some xenophobic medical personnel, political posture, or institutionalized systemic procedure—and due to the avoidable, unnecessary, and preventable nature of their illnesses and treatment, their experiences are the consequence and product of structural violence.

In his book, *Violence: Reflections on a National Epidemic*, James Gilligan explains structural violence as "the increased rates of death and disability suffered by those who occupy the bottom rungs of society, as contrasted with the relatively lower death rates experienced by those who are above them" (1996, 192). One such example of this is the disease of (standard) Tuberculosis, a malady that has been around since the time of the ancient Egyptian Pharaohs, yet access to diagnosis and a low-cost treatment developed back in 1940s remains an enduring stumbling block today in poor countries. (This example does not endeavor to include the newer strains of multidrug-resistant tuberculosis [MDR TB], or extensively drug-resistant TB [XDR-TB], or totally drug-resistant tuberculosis [TDR-TB] forms.) Tuberculosis is a prime example of structural violence in that our modern society's current course of one six-month standard TB treatment drugs cost approximately $20—yet in 2008, there were an estimated 9.4 million new TB cases, and 1.8 million TB deaths (WHO, 2010). The current African "blight" of drug-resistant forms of tuberculosis, both XDR-TB and MDR-TB, are ravaging HIV and other immuno-compromised populations. Since PPD (purified protein derivative) TB testing doesn't seek the Mycobacterium tuberculosis, but rather only tests if the patient's immune system is combating the bacteria—many HIV patients lack sufficient immune activity to either fight the infection or properly respond as "positive" to the PPD test (AIDSMEDS, 2012). Therefore, perfunctory TB testing is not as dependable in HIV-positive people with compromised immune systems, so many times a diagnosis of TB will not be made until (further) acute symptoms arise, and/or more sophisticated testing like X-rays, sputum or blood tests are performed. In Paul Farmer's *Infections and Inequalities: The Modern Plagues* book published in 1999, he cited five assertions that "hold true" for drug-resistant tuberculosis as well as global HIV strategies: (1) effective treatment cannot be solely the province of wealthy countries, as TB remains, along with AIDS, the "leading infectious cause of adult death in the world today"; (2) cost effectiveness cannot be the only measure by which public health interventions are evaluated as any costly intervention that serves destitute and sickly populations is diametrically opposed to profit-making corporate welfare goals; (3) research in developing countries has to include social justice initiatives because, as Farmer notes, "poor people are excellent lab rats but unlikely patients" concerning first-world diagnostics on third-world data collection subjects; (4) more effective prevention strategies are needed as the "education as the only vaccine" tactic is "neither accurate nor wise"; (5) the notion of "limited resources" should not be silently accepted as verbatim now. Farmer insists that there is no data to prove that there are currently scarcer fiscal resources available today—a time when there are more, not less—effective therapies for diseases than ever before (xxiii–xxvi). Clearly, more equitable access to efficacious medical treatments is a necessary fundamental step in reducing these life-threatening infectious diseases.

Along the same vein, difficulties that can make a healthy delivery and complication-free pregnancy precarious, or even fatal, for women can be structural—and yet so are issues that marginalize or place a "token" emphasis women's health and/or that constrain a woman's ability and authority to seek healthcare for herself. Hence structural violence limits a person's life, quality of life, and inflicts unnecessary physical pain and mental anguish.

GENDER-BASED VIOLENCE AND FEMINIST THEORY

Feminist scholars note that: "Gender is a social construction and to specify one's gender automatically entails questions about relations of race, class and political power" (Meintjes et al. 2001, 5). Nonetheless gender remains at the core of most societies' organizing principals "affecting rights, responsibilities, self-efficacy, exposure to risk, and access to healthcare" (Richter 2015). A feminist research epistemology was employed in this research since feminism's most engaging and persuasive epistemological insight is deemed by noted feminist scholars (Doucet and Mauthner 2006; Lennon and Whitford 1994) as the conjoining of constructs of knowledge and power. Even so, Sandra Harding has remarked that the rationality of "standpoint epistemologists" (and feminists who exercise this theory) "start thought with marginalized lives," and subsequently "takes everyday life as problematic" (1993, 15)—thus, this research utilizes correlations between power inequities and health/welfare entrées.

In a no-win paradoxical catch-22, Ghanaian women can find themselves as social scapegoats in both hardship and success, and be keen to avoid any and all missteps in that: "She must not fall below expectation; neither must she rise above it" (Ter Haar 2007, 83). In this shooting gallery fête, whichever woman dares to raise her head up financially or educationally (above men and other women)—she will be rapidly and categorically shot down. And her dramatic expulsion will forever hold sway as a "warning" portent to other Ghanaian women who might deign to challenge the status quo. Additionally, any outward behavior(s) that may be considered "eccentric" as in the cases of "those who mutter to themselves, or are regarded as inquisitive, meddlesome, garrulous, and cantankerous" (Adinkrah 2004, 336) can also incite social friction, accusations, and open conflict. Even so, perhaps most disturbing and disheartening is how successful women or intelligent young female students—dubbed as "outspoken," "domineering" or "assertive" or "bewitched"—remain undeniably the easiest potential prey. Obviously, these practices hamstring many women's initiatives to increase their economic productivity, raise their educational standing, and/or promote or 'show off' their public station. Undoubtedly, these toxic "social indictments" generate not only distrust, strained familial relations, and cultural dissention—but also widespread inequitable economic development, and local (Region-based) and national fiscal insecurity.

Early studies of witchcraft among the Dagomba revealed that the majority of the people who were accused of practicing witchcraft were women, and many of them traveled to the shrines to "prove their innocence or to cleanse themselves of the curse of witchcraft" (Parker 2006, 374). The predominance of literature on witchcraft demonstrates that women bear an inequitable burden due to gender-based discrimination. In his study, West African Traditional Religion, Kofi Asare Opoku, states what the society takes for granted that "witches are usually women, although one occasionally encounters confessed witches who are children" (1978, 142). Taking a critical approach of the general belief that many of the witches are women, Ghanaian theologian Mercy Amba Oduyoye has argued that since older women tend to be respected, sometimes the idea that they are suspected to be witches is stated in folktales which portray women as wicked witches (Oduyoye 1995). In the Asante region, witch-finding cults composed primarily of men were called Aberewa (old woman), but the men—who according to local traditions should have been witches themselves to detect it in another person—were considered to be "good" witches. It was generally thought that "witches were women who work against the unity and coherence of community, and who do not seek the good of others or actively care for others" (Oduyoye 1995, 121). When it comes to women then, the general neutrality that is often assumed about witchcraft (that it can be used for good or evil) is put aside because it is believed that women use their own witchcraft in an anti-social manner. In 1988, educational materials indicated that witchcraft could be used for good or ill; therefore there is good witchcraft and bad witchcraft (GES 1988). The tradition of putting the burden of negative witchcraft on women has continued in postcolonial Ghana as some women have been accused of being witches because they were highly educated or successful in business (Oduyoye 1995 and Amoah 1990). It was not unexpected that gender proved a significant matter in our conversations with the women of Gnani.

It was clear to us from our interviews in 2007, 2008, 2015, and other previous interviews that witchcraft and the decision to move suspected witches to a special village, like the trokosi, raises important gender questions. The idea of witches' village with a large population whose inhabitants were mostly women, suggested that gender was a major factor in witchcraft beliefs, accusation, and punishment. Several of the women think they were accused because they did not have anyone to support them. Their husbands had died, and from the way they talked about it, one got the impression that they felt that if their husbands were alive, they would have supported them. It has hard in these cases to know if their husbands would actually have come to their defense, especially if they subscribed to the logic and beliefs of witchcraft prevalent in these localities and the structure of patrilineal society. But there is something to be said about the fact that many of the women pointed out that their husbands were deceased at the time of the accusation.

Alice, who identified as a Baptist Christian and has lived at the village for 23 years, emphasized the gender dimension of witchcraft discourses and practice. She was accused of killing her brother-in-law through witchcraft. In our conversation with her, she indicated that men have also been accused of being witches and reminded us that some of the residents of the village were men who themselves were accused of being witches. When we asked why it is the case that even in a village where it is estimated that there are several hundred residents, most of the residents are women accused, she said that women were accused because they are "weaker than men," a reference to the fact that fewer women would be able and/or willing to challenge a man or a group of people in what could turn out to be a prolonged struggle. However, she rejected the view that women were bad people or used their powers to do evil as it was alleged in the allegations. This incidence reminded Bongmba of a similar occurrence he had witnessed in his native Wimbum area of Cameroon, where several individuals were accused of using witchcraft to kill a member of the community. Several of them were women and they were forced into exile. Yet when the residents of the community approached one man—who was accused along with the other women—he deftly loaded up his gun and told them that he was waiting for the person who would come and try to remove him out of his house. Not so coincidentally, no one ever challenged the man, and he was never exiled.

Alice seemed to be a very informed woman, but when we asked if women can do something about these accusations, she thought that there is really no hope that women can do something about their fate because no one will listen. We asked if they have talked to state and local officials and asked them to do something about the situation and she said they often do but no one has come to help them address the situation. We asked if local elected politicians have heard their plight and she told us that they even come to the witches' village to campaign for their votes and make promises—yet they never keep those promises. Asked if they have considered starting a movement that would challenge those politicians and demand that they do something that would stop the practice of exiling people to witches' villages, she said it was an idea they should consider because they certainly do not want their children and grandchildren to be exiled in the future.

If one were to further contemplate such an assumption of action/non-action, one would realize that these women would need to lead substantial sociocultural, spiritual, and economic reforms counter to traditions that have existed for over a hundred years. Nonetheless, many of the women lack the representation, legal acumen (judicial, civil, and/or criminal), overall good health and nourishment, educational skills, and resources necessary to mount such an effort. There is a case that demonstrates how complex this issue is in contemporary Ghana as it is in other African communities where witchcraft has turned violent which makes our question or suggestion that individual women do something about it sound mostly academic. Let us reflect on the case of another woman we called Abena, who was accused of killing her nephew through witchcraft. The nephew was on his way to school, became ill and eventually died in the hospital. The nephew died even before health-care workers had time to diagnose his illness. But Abena was accused and she claimed that this was done because her husband had died and there was no one to defend her. Abena insisted that if her late husband were alive, he would have defended her. Abena's son, a locally elected assemblyman, attempted to defend her (stating that the 'medicine' she drank proved her innocence), but the villagers continued to profess her guilt. In an ensuing struggle to defend his mother, the son shot two people and was sentenced to life imprisonment (albeit deprived of legal counsel). Abena was summarily captured and conveyed to the witches' village. We asked if the police had spoken to her (or anyone else) to gather evidence and she said no one had ever contacted her. She also believed that had her son received a fair trial, he (and Abena) would have been vindicated through pleas of self-defense. Asked if the local chiefs and the paramount chief have been involved in seeking adjudication, Abena was unsure if any traditional elders had been notified of the incident. This case harrowingly illustrates the extreme subjugation and vulnerability of women.

Considering gendered "glass ceilings" and socially acceptable gender roles and taboos, Akrong has argued:

> Witchcraft is often used as one of the ways of enforcing these rigid gender roles, especially for women in order to keep them from 'gate-crushing' into roles traditionally reserved for men alone. The association of witchcraft with evil makes it a very dangerous tag to put on anybody, because once a person is identified as a witch, she becomes a social outcast, who loses all her human rights. This is the main reason why in certain parts of northern Ghana women accused of witchcraft stay in witch villages. (2007)

In yet another instance, on the eve of the millennium, there was a meningitis outbreak in northern Ghana of 1,396 cases that led to 63 fatalities. In March of 1997, street-vigilante violence was directed against several women in northern Ghana on suspicion that they were responsible for the spread of what was diagnosed as cerebrospinal meningitis (CSM) (Roberts 2000). During the epidemic, it was reported that women were killed and others were sent to witches' villages. Violence has been associated with witchcraft in South Africa, and as in Ghana, the victims were murdered (Schnoebelen 2009). Adinkrah has documented 40 reported witch murders in Ghana between 1980 and 2012—recording 31 of the 40 victims as female (Adinkrah 2015).

The negative effect of witchcraft beliefs on women have been documented in other places in Africa. Bongmba has argued that in the Wimbum community of the northwest province in Cameroon, tʉ (witchcraft) can be understood as gender discourse because most of the victims of the accusations are women (2001). Diane Lyons has argued that in Dela area of Cameroon "witchcraft is part of a complex of social practices which reproduce the perception that women as witches are antisocial and impermanent . . . the representation of women as witches is a means. . . to restrict women's access to key resources. . ." (1998, 346). These two examples from Cameroon mirror research that documents the victimization of women through witchcraft accusations. As Professor Dzodzi Tsikata of the University of Ghana explained, "women are expected to be submissive so once you start to be outspoken in your views or even successful in your trade, people assume you must be possessed" (Whitaker 2012). One such reprehensible case was reported in 2012, when a 17-year-old high school girl was sent to a witches' camp by members of her community because she was exceptionally intelligent. The young girl was accused of bewitching and "stealing the intelligence" of her classmates and banished to the Gambaga Witches Camp in the Northern Region. Additionally, young Ghanaian children are socialized into witchcraft by being utilized as perpetrators of "punitive practices" such as the stoning of accused women, indelibly affecting children's respect for women, as men are never lynched (Ter Haar 2007, 82).

Inclusively and/or exclusively, the indefensible violence against innocent females as "witches" can be considered the product(s) of any variety of social impetuses, religious influences, and/or metal phobias, including, but not limited to: Misogyny (the dislike of, contempt for, or ingrained prejudice against women) or Patriarchy (a social organization marked by the supremacy of the father in the clan or family, the legal dependence of wives and children, and the reckoning of descent and inheritance in the male line; and control by men of a disproportionately large share of power); Male Chauvinism (who patronizes, disparages, or otherwise denigrates females in the belief that they are inferior to males and thus deserving of less than equal treatment or benefit); Bigotry (stubborn and complete intolerance of any creed, belief, or opinion that differs from one's own); Gynophobia (fear of women); Ageism and/or Gerontophobia (a hatred or fear of the elderly); or even Caligynephobia/Venustraphobia (the fear of beautiful women in particular) (Merriam-Webster 2015). People with these phobias or aberrant can feel dread, panic, terror, and feelings of hatred or inferiority towards women.

According to "Witchcraft in a modern age: broken communities and recalcitrant stigma," a December 2015 report by the OHCHR, women accused of witchcraft among the populations displaced by the recent ethnic and religious conflict in the Central African Republic are primarily older women abandoned by their families "because of the burden they represent" and left with no support in their community, or "girls as young as five years old are accused of having inherited the sorcery gene from their mothers or their neighbors," or enterprising women who are said to be earning a living "too decent to be natural in times like these" (OHCHR 2015, 1). Human Rights Division of the UN Integrated Missions for the Stabilization in Central African Republic carried out a series of activities to raise awareness about women's and girls' rights. The Office has also been advocating with decision and law makers for the prevention of gender-based violence, and reminding the authorities of their obligation to protect individuals from mob justice and investigate and prosecute perpetrators of such crimes. The local office of the Human Rights Division in Kaga Bandoro and the Association for Sustainable Development in Rural Areas in CAR organised an informational session on violence related to witchcraft accusations at the internally displaced persons' camp of Bamou, three kilometers south of Kaga Bandoro that houses some 2,723 people. "Often, when an elderly and destitute woman asks a young person for food and if that young person happens to fall ill, the population usually immediately accuses her of being a witch," said one woman attending the session.

Women and girls accused of witchcraft suffer the most cruel, inhuman, and degrading treatment that strips them of all the human dignity they had left. They are mostly the victims of mob justice characterized by stoning, the forced administration of poisonous substances, flogging, and burying people alive. Victims have also been exposed to flames after being tied and bound, or forced to pay fines in the form of money, cattle, or their agricultural produce. Others whose lives are spared are victims of arbitrary arrest and detention. During the session, facilitators stressed that mob justice is not only contrary to human rights law, but also prohibited under Central African law. "No one has the right to take justice in their own hands," said the human rights facilitators. "Together let us turn to the principle of '*Zo Kwe Zo*' (Any human being is a human being), which is the motto of the Central African people." The Penal Code of the Central African Republic contains provisions against quackery and witchcraft. Articles 149 and 150 state that a fine of up to 1,000,000 CFA francs (approximately $ 1,670 U.S. dollars) and a sentence between five and ten years imprisonment will be imposed on whomever is found guilty of practicing witchcraft which results in bodily harm to their victim; or a life sentence of forced labour if those practices lead to the death of their victim (OHCHR 2015).

In fact, these settlements are known as "*pwaanyankura-foango*," a Mampruli term meaning "old ladies section" (Kirby 2012, 199 and Tetzlaff 2015). There are, conceivably, a myriad of ethical dilemmas specifically poised at feminist fieldwork and quasi-ethnographical participatory methodologies, due in part to its contemporary nature, thus it functions in dynamic academic, participatory, ethical, and observational arenas.

AGEISM, ELDER ABUSE, AND ADVOCACY

Irrefutably, the vast majority of inhabitants in witches' villages and main victims of witchcraft allegations are female, and in particular, older, widowed, and uneducated women. Treated with rejection and contempt, some of these post-menopausal Ghanaian women (past child-bearing years) voluntarily exile themselves to a witches' village rather than suffer the public degradation and physical battery that would—with a high probable likelihood—eventually come to bear whenever some misfortune, hardship, or death visited the woman's village. So how do these sentiments coexist within a society that (overtly) values, and even readily esteems, the wisdom that comes with old age? As Sjaak van der Geest, emeritus professor of Medical Anthropology at the University of Amsterdam, revealed the word "old" has a positive connotation in Ghana (e.g., "*I am old*" translates as "*I have grown*") however the "borders between respect and hatred, admiration and envy, affection and fear prove porous" (van der Geest 2005). This ambiguous interplay between respect, jealousy, fear, and distrust form a quixotic composition. As van der Geest explains here:

> Their spiritual power is sometimes appreciated as wisdom, the fruit of lifelong experience. At other times that spiritual power is denounced as witchcraft.

Theologically these statements sound confusing and contradictory. From a sociological point of view, however, they make sense. They express the basic ambivalence of young people towards the old. On one hand there is respect, a cultural code which is almost 'natural': one regards with awe and admiration what came before. On the other, old people engender resentment because of their overbearing attitude and their refusal to 'go.' The fact that young people die while old people remain alive is a reversal of the natural order and reeks of witchcraft. (2005, 462)

Civil society groups must step up efforts to demystify the myth surrounding the age old concept of witchcraft which seems not to have any empirical basis. For water, the inhabitants of the Kukuo camp walk three miles each day to the River Otti, struggling back uphill with heavy pots of water. It's an intolerable way for an elderly woman to live, but it's a life they are prepared to endure so long as they are safe. They survive by collecting firewood, selling little bags of peanuts or working in nearby farms. A 2012 ActionAid report stated that more than 70 percent of residents in Ghana's Kukuo camp were accused and banished after their husbands died—implying that witchcraft allegations are a way of empowering disgruntled or impoverished family members to take control of the widow's property (Whitaker 2012). Professor Dzodzi Tsikata of the University of Ghana explained that the camps "are a dramatic manifestation of the status of women in Ghana. Older women become a target because they are no longer useful to society" (Whitaker 2012, 1). Moreover, by no stretch of the imagination, most cultural practices in northern Ghana could be viewed as unfavorable to women. These traditional practices can include outmoded widowhood/mourning rites, and inheritance properties of their parents including land ownership. The opening statement of the U.N.'s June 2014 report, "U.N. Findings Flag Violence, Abuse of Older Women Accused of Witchcraft" was: "Did you know violence and abuse against elderly women, the world's fastest growing demographic group, range from sexual violence, property grabbing, financial abuse and increasingly, extreme violence against older women accused of witchcraft?" (UN 2014). The report continues on to note that: "Witchcraft accusations that are used to justify extreme violence against older women are reported in 41 African and Asian countries including Burkina Faso, Cameroon, India, Kenya, Malawi, Nepal, and Tanzania. Older widows are often those most at risk" (UN 2014, 1). According to U.N. Secretary-General Ban Ki-moon, older women are at particular risk due to widespread discriminatory attitudes and practices, and urged countries to enact and enforce stronger laws and strategies to address all aspects of this under-acknowledged social, public health, and human rights issue and designated June 15 as "World Elder Abuse Awareness Day" under UN resolution 66/127 (UN 2014). The UN World Health Organization stated that abuse is under-reported by as much as 80 percent, and that the global population of people aged 60 years and older is expected to more than double (from 542 million in 1995 to about 1.2 billion in 2025) thus the segment of elderly persons (60 years+) in the total population increased from 9 percent in 1994 to 12 percent in 2014, and is projected to attain 21 percent by 2050 (UN 2014).

Zakari goes on to explain that from a Ghanaian insight, nothing more than the visible onset of the body's natural aging processes (i.e., wrinkles, sagging skin, age-spots, purpura rashes, cracked skin) can be cause for witchcraft allegations:

> From a Ghanaian perception, witchcraft is the art of leaving one's body in the night to fly about, and turn to magic, and catch people's souls, which are then turned into animals by the use of spells, charms, conjuring, and/or new spirits. Witches and wizards—after being accused—are sent to the witches' camps for trials of their powers. However, before a man or a woman [can] be called a wizard or a witch, something unfortunate would have happened in the area he or she lives. *First and more famously, the aged are accused as their bodies have turned naturally wrinkled, and they are not far from been accused of being witches and wizards.* Other accusations are generated from certain dreams of individuals that seemed to be badly interpreted. Also, envy and jealousy [from other people] can lead to witchcraft accusation. In the northern region of Ghana, this practice is widespread. (2015)

Thus, old, disabled, poor, or widowed women are often subjected to witchcraft accusations for any number of gratuitous grounds, including: surviving a husband; older women are seen as having "little value because they are no longer economically or biologically productive in the household"; unwanted characteristics such as red eyes (oftentimes caused by prolonged exposure to cooking fires), living alone, or eccentric behavior; miscarrying or losing a child, according to USA-based nonprofit HelpAge USA (2015, 1). The NGO HelpAge has worked in 90 villages, training community members as paralegal advisers to provide support and advice on land, inheritance, and marriage rights in 20,000 cases, with nearly half of the disputes concerning inheritance and land rights for older women between 2004 and 2008 (2015). These inheritance-based accusations essentially cut the accused off, not only from any familial obligations of shelter, feeding, and care, but also "any future inheritance" competitions (Daswani 2010, 451).

On a positive note, HelpAge boasts results worthy of replication: Their community interventions have ushered in a 99 percent reduction in the killing of older women in the areas where they and their partners are actively running projects, a significant reduction in disputes over land rights, inheritance and matrimonial issues, as well as a 30 percent improvement in living conditions of older women (HelpAge 2015). While Ghanaian law criminalizes harmful mourning rites, widows (especially in the Upper West region) are forced to undergo indigenous rites such as a one-year period of mourning, tying ropes and padlocks around the widow's waist, forced sitting (next to deceased spouse) until his burial, solitary confinement, forced starvation, shaving of the widow's hair, and/or smearing clay on her body—should she engage in prosperous economic activity after her husband's death, she may be regarded as adulterous, the cause of his death, or condemned as a witch (U.S. Dept. of State 2011).

In the end, these tragic beliefs do nothing more than stifle the country's economic development, and dumb-down young Ghanaian female intellectuals—striking down potential future industry leaders, political trailblazers, and scholastic educators—before they even initiate any attempt at an achievement.

Chapter Six

Facing Forward

We do note that the controversies that have been generated by the existence of these villages in the twenty-first century reflect the dynamic nature of witchcraft discourses and alleged practices. The women, who have long known that something was amiss, now acknowledge abandonment, false accusations, exile, and/or threats of violence. The Ghanaian government and international NGOs view occurrences surrounding the northern Ghana witches' villages as a violation of human rights and freedoms, as well as the failure of the state to apply the law to address issues that affect the wellbeing of a large number of Ghanaians. This is a significant shift from merely considering witchcraft discourses as a passé or outmoded discourse, but rather seeing it as a contemporary engagement in the dialectics and dynamics of social existence in the post-colony.

In this chapter we will then explore dialectics and dynamics of witchcraft in contemporary Ghanaian society, and address how the current national media content serves to eradicate, indoctrinate, or cultivate witchcraft beliefs via TV, radio, films, as well as other social media mechanisms. It is in this chapter's review that we will also consider legal, constitutional, and human rights perspectives that call for legal intervention, enforcement, and prosecution of discrimination against people on the suspicion that there are witches. We will also address the dilemmas of contemporary lawmakers, police, human rights activists, and members of the legal profession who grapple with questionable testimonies, dubious circumstantial evidence, and arbitrary accusations. We will conclude this final chapter by addressing the implications of our findings, and offering ten recommendations that each draw from our research, medical data, and examination of the spiritual, medical, and economic conditions of the Gnani residents.

THE DIALECTICS AND DYNAMICS OF WITCHCRAFT IN CONTEMPORARY GHANA

The dialogues with the residents of Gnani witches' village reflect the dialectics of a community in transition where the old lingers and the residents are surrounded by the outside world that looks on with shock but also debates what is appropriate. The dialogue on witchcraft in the Gnani area started a long time ago, and for reasons which today some people question, the locals in the village determined that things just don't happen and in the case of misfortune the causal agent is often human. The members of the society who were believed to have the power to inflict harm and cause the death of others in the community were singled out, exiled, or isolated. The consensus at some point was that if such a thing happened, exile was a suitable way to purge the guilty party from the community. They were alleged to have killed or caused harm to someone—yet the community spared their lives; some would argue it exemplifies a "quintessential religious act" against the act of manslaughter. However, the accused are deprived of having a fair and public hearing which could safeguard people against unlawful and/or arbitrary restriction or dispossession of their rights to life and liberty. According to the United Nations Human Rights Office of the High Commissioner's International Covenant on Civil and Political Rights (ICCPR), the definition of 'fair trial' consists of voluminous issues, nevertheless we will mention, in an abridged fashion, three critical sections that directly pertain to our research:

> 1.) All persons shall be equal before the courts and tribunals. In the determination of any criminal charge against him, or of his rights and obligations in a suit at law, everyone shall be entitled to a fair and public hearing by a *competent, independent and impartial tribunal* established by law; 2.) Everyone charged with a criminal offence shall have the *right to be presumed innocent* until proved guilty according to law; 3.) In the determination of any criminal charge against him, everyone shall be entitled to the following minimum guarantees, in full equality: (a) To be *informed promptly and in detail in a language which he understands* of the nature and cause of the charge against him. (United Nations Human Rights Office of the High Commissioner ICCPR, Article 14, section 1–3)

But the times have changed and the dynamics too have shifted. While many still believe in witchcraft in Ghana, there is no generally accepted public consensus about what to think of it. While many still see it as anti-social behavior, and thus classify them as negative actions which should be sanctioned, there is a growing body of opinion from people who are not so sure what to do with the idea and belief of witchcraft in Ghana today. Other people in some African countries think that there is such a power that can be deployed for evil purposes, but there are aspects of this power that are neutral or even benign (Bongmba 2001). But in the main, many still think and would agree with Kofi Asare Opoku (1978) that witches have and deploy esoteric power for their own schemes. One cannot understand these discourses and the interpretation of these powers as a national phenomenon because to do so would be to miss the local sensitivities to the debate in different parts of a country like Ghana. While someone in another part of the country may choose to adopt a completely scientific outlook, other people in different parts of the country may not compartmentalize their lives that way. Trusting that scientific information is relevant to them does not negate a belief in the powers of the occult or witchcraft. Therefore, thinking of both offers them alternative ways of arriving at meaning when faced with complex questions and things they consider mysterious. This debate on different forms of causality goes back to the earliest literature on witchcraft in African Studies (Opoku 1978, and DeBrunner 1961).

If one were to follow the literature, one could argue that in many ways not much has changed in the Gnani, as the emphasis on witchcraft (a belief that people have the ability to utilize it to kill someone) remains. Thus there is a very traditional view to witchcraft. This would be a misunderstanding of the situation because from our interviews, it is clear that the women (who themselves are victims) are raising new inquiries about their condition. The fact that many of them feel "weak" as women, or claim that they think it was easy for the community to bring charges against them as widowers, indicates that the dynamics of witchcraft reflect contemporary questions (Gescheire 1996). There is also no doubt that accusations (based solely on the dreams that individuals have had, especially children) raise new questions about the role of dreams (or even if one were to broaden it)—the fear(s) and imagination(s) of certain individuals raise new questions about witchcraft. The fact that a young boy's dream is evidence enough to convict and condemn someone into exile demonstrates how the "rules of evidence" in witchcraft may have waned rather that intensified in contemporary witchcraft discourses, leaving observers to wonder if anything has changed at all in witchcraft beliefs (Assimeng 1989). Yet the Gnani stories do highlight a very individual dimension of witchcraft. The accusations are about individual people doing something which people consider antisocial. These accounts point to a different type of psychodynamic activities. In our interviews we did not hear any stories of people banding together in a witch society to cause misfortune. None of the people we interviewed talked of witches attending a society where human flesh was consumed. We think it might not be appropriate to claim that there are no witch Sabbaths in Ghana or that people do not meet together with guilds as they allegedly used to do in the past (Akrong 2007). We do not know why most of the cases in the Gnani area emphasize death, illness, or seem to allude only to causing harm to younger children when elsewhere in Ghana Elom Dovlo argues: "powers attributed to 'witches' include the ability to inflict material loss through fire, theft, crop failure," and "poor spending," as well as, "sterility, impotence or disease such as leprosy" (2007, 68).

The seriousness with which the Ghanaian community is addressing the question of witches' villages cannot be called into question. During the last decade many stake holders, politicians, jurist, human rights activists, religious leaders, and non-governmental organizations have framed the debate as a major human rights issue and brought into the debate the legal and statutory provisions of the Ghanaian legal system. While confining people in the past away from their place of residence for using witchcraft might have been acceptable or might have seemed prudent to some people, it is no longer the case today. In 2010, according to the Southern Sector Youth and Women's Empowerment Network (SOSYWEN), Justice Emile Short of the Commission on Human rights and Administrative Justice (CHRAJ) stated unequivocally:

> As a statutory human rights institution charged with the responsibility for preventing and redressing human rights violations, we are interested in safeguarding the rights of all sections of our society. For that reason, the treatment meted out to suspected witches, which violates human rights, is of grave concern to us. Apart from losing their liberty to live freely in their natural homes and communities, their rights to dignity, to own property, and to freedom of movement and expression are all curtailed. We strongly recommend that the government extends its social services e.g. LEAP, to cater for these women in the "witches" camps. (SOSYWEN 2011)

For these women and the few men who have also been accused, the question is what or where is home. From the first time we read about the witches' camps in Ghana and watched Allison Berg's film, "Witches in Exile," and a later film, "The Witches of Gambaga," most people have said that it is cruel to confine these women to these villages and we agree. Surely no person in the right mind would want to live in this place. Many of us have criticized the Ghanaian government for turning away from the disruptions which many of these women face and the horrible conditions of the villages in which they live. For many people, the most pressing concern is the violations of their personal freedoms and disregard for their rights. Those rights are violated with impunity to a large extent, as we have argued, because they are women.

We spoke with some people in Accra who suggested that the international attention the women living in witches' villages have received has made them cause célébré and they believed that their removal from these villages would make them somehow forfeit this covered global attention. Without being judgmental of individual opinion, we consider this proposition as preposterous. First, these women are unmistakably victims of a belief system that calls for comprehensive rethinking. Secondly, condemned witches have immeasurably suffered under marginalized conditions for decades—not a sought-after position any person in a stable mental condition would seek to voluntarily embrace. Third, whatever short-lived attention these women have been afforded is fleeting, as the global media attention they had previously experienced in 2012–2014 seems to be waning rather than waxing.

CULTURES OF ERADICATION OR CULTIVATION?

However it is interesting to note here that ordinary people everywhere—in every stressed corner of society—resort to some formulary of "magic" as an emotional coping mechanism. Any form of mass manipulation and social control that leads to an illusionary or synthetic form of happiness can be construed as magic. American civilization's "juju" can take the forms of religious fervor, Internet or iPhone addiction, work obsession, alcohol, money, and TV—all mixed with a liberal dose of Prozac or some other prescription drug(s). Indeed, any source of counterfeit gratification or bogus absolution that people turn to in order to help numb "the pain of reality" (e.g., personal failure, sexual impotence, inexplicable misfortune) can be interpreted as a supernatural fairytale. Back in 1843, German economist and Communist political philosopher Karl Marx famously stated in his *Critique of Hegel's Philosophy of Right: "Die Religion . . . ist das Opium des Volkes,"* speaking to religion as mere foolishness of the *hoi polloi,* and "the sigh of the oppressed creature, the heart of a heartless world, and the soul of soulless conditions. It is the opium of the people" (Marx 1843, 378–379). There is an indisputable and marked "parallel acceptance" of medical sciences and spiritual healing innately woven into the collective modern-American Christian psyche. Oftentimes modern-day rationales falsely presuppose that first-world development equates to secular, technology- and science-based convictions. Nothing could be further from the truth. To be sure, the Western world (replete with all of its twenty-first century "New Age" religions) is not obligated to any singular secular justification(s) in science, medicine, technology, or elsewhere—nor is it as distant from Ghana's supernatural belief systems as it may keenly (or readily) surmise.

Yet there is customarily something behind every defamatory accusation: an easy, vulnerable target; jealousy; superstition; or sometimes even a mistaken or misplaced conviction. "The belief in witchcraft is pervasive in Ghana. We don't have exact statistics, but recent studies show that about 90 per cent of Ghanaians believe in witches and in witchcraft," stated ActionAid's Kwesi Tawiah-Benjamin (Dunn 2015, 1). As Adinkrah noted, the Ghanaian public experiences a lifelong "socialization into witchcraft ideology" via popular Ghanaian music, television shows, popular dramas in theaters and concerts, newspapers, DVD films, broadcast religious sermons, the Internet (disseminates 'witchcraft-related' crimes, news, and accounts on Ghana-based websites like Ghanatoday.com, Ghanaweb.com, Ghanacrunch.com, Ghanareview.com), radio shows, and even Akan proverbs (2015, 119). "Radio may have a greater impact on teaching about witchcraft than television and video," explained Adinkrah, as there is a greater accessibility to public radio programming with over 50 stations and 12.5 million radio and wireless sets in the country as opposed to the ownership of more-expensive TV sets and services (Adinkrah 2015, 119). Ter Haar concurs with Adinkrah's comments on the Ghanaian media's effect on the general public:

> They actually foster the belief in witchcraft by carrying stories of witchcraft confessions and particularly of pastors exorcising people of witchcraft (often with pictures). This is also a popular theme of video films, mostly produced in Nigeria, that sell in Ghana and are shown to the public in video theaters but also on Ghanaian television. (Ter Haar 2007, 72)

Many of these nationally distributed media outlets warn Ghanaians about the ever-present threat and obsessed conspiracies of modern witches, be-witchings, witch groups, a witch's working *modus operandi*, and anti-witch-craft solutions and/or prescriptions. The singular repetitious onslaught of imagery and machinations of witchcraft has myself and other members of our medical team to boycott most of the popular TV evening 'soap opera' dramas, and many newspapers while in Ghana, as the principal topic is, more times than not, revolving around a case of bewitching gone bad.

Indeed, new studies show that witchcraft themes in the Ghanaian film industry are more popular than ever. With the burgeoning growth of neigh-boring Nollywood, Nigeria's take on Hollywood and the third largest global film producer with a $200,000,000 annual industry—Ghana's Akan-language Kumawood (taken from Kumasi, the capital of the Ashanti Region in Ghana) is booming while English-speaking "Glamour" movies decline in popularity (Meyer 2015 and Yamoah 2014). These newly produced Kuma-wood films "resonate culturally and nationally with Ghanaians" (Yamoah 2014, 161). And while these locally produced films definitively spur the development of a unique domestic art form, local culture(s), national audi-ences, and commercial markets, the effects of a deeper entrenchment of witchcraft phenomena into Ghanaian media products may only serve to rein-force and further engender witchcraft mythology and ideology.

According to the not-for-profit U.K.-based group Witchcraft and Human Rights Information Network (WHRIN) Executive Director, Gary Foxcroft:

> Laws and policies alone will not put a stop to these horrific forms of human rights abuses. In addition to wide-spread awareness raising activities to demys-tify the perceived supernatural powers of albinos, government agencies need

to look at the role that Nollywood films are playing in promoting these beliefs. Such films, which are widely viewed in the region and often feature themes relating to witchcraft, help spread such superstitious beliefs. (Witchcraft and Human Rights Information Network 2013, 1)

One new film, "The Cursed Ones," by Ghanaian-born Nana Obiri Yeboa, tells the story of a disillusioned reporter and a young reformed Pastor attempting to save the life of a child accused of witchcraft (BBC News 2015). The film, which hopes to dispel local violence against condemned 'witches' is being shown in London as part of a festival hosted by The Royal African Society. The time has come for more attention to be paid to this emerging issue and for greater efforts to be made to find solutions to it.

LEGAL AND CONSTITUTIONAL MATTERS

Ghana is a constitutional democracy including an authoritative presidency and a unicameral (single legislative chamber) 275-seat parliament. In Ghana, there stand Constitutional Acts, legislative laws/powers, chieftaincy instruments, and other mechanisms that govern the management of the national institution. Current research conducted by the National House of Chiefs in collaboration with the Ministry of Chieftaincy and Traditional Affairs (MCTA) with support from the United States Agency for International Development (USAID), revealed that "witchcraft is predominant in the Northern Region, widowhood rites in the Upper East Region, and FGM in the Upper West Region" in Ghana (Development News Africa 2015). According to Article 272(c) of the 1992 Fourth Republican Constitution of Ghana the National House of Chiefs is to, "undertake an evaluation of traditional customs and usages with a view to eliminating those customs and usages that are socially harmful" (Ghana Constitution 1992). Furthermore, the national constitution stipulates under Article 26 (2) that: "All customary practices which dehumanise or are injurious to the physical and mental well-being of a person are prohibited," and Article 39 (2) goes on to pledge that: "The State shall ensure that appropriate customary and cultural values are adopted and developed as an integral part of the growing needs of the society as a whole, and in particular that traditional practices which are injurious to health and wellbeing of the person are abolished" (Ghana Constitution 1992). Ghana's Chieftaincy Act of 2008 Act 759 Section 50 states that: "Where a Traditional Council determines that the customary law which is in force within its area is uncertain or consider it desirable that it should be modified or assimilated by the common law, the council shall make representation on the matter to the House of Chiefs in the Region" (2008). Therefore Ghanaian law(s) unmistakably allow traditional authorities the leverage to alter any and all customs and/or traditions that are considered injurious or detrimental to their people.

Therefore, given the multifaceted complexities of this social, fiscal, and gender-based enigma, what can be done to impeach and thwart unjust future witchcraft accusations in Ghana? Although many educated Ghanaians tend not to believe in such phenomena, they acknowledge the belief as part of their cultural background, noting that "it's difficult for outsiders to understand, but African daily life relies heavily on the spirit world, for good or evil" (Nkatazo 2006). Other researchers argue that the expeditious expulsion of witchcraft belief systems from Africa would further daunt emergent "organic" African jurisprudence, hinder rural conflict resolution, and create spiritual insecurity (Ashforth 2015; Ter Haar 2007). Our field experience and transdisciplinary research would argue that while it would be unwise to espouse legal and/or social policies that undermine collective justice (or common people constituting a fundamental politico-economic grouping) grassroots efforts of self-governance in Ghana—likewise, it would prove imprudent to not hold police and justice institutions accountable for such patent human rights abuses.

Another salient human rights' concern is the "witches" loss of voting rights during national elections. According to one report from *Modern Ghana*: "Most women in Gambaga camp just like other witches camp, they are always denied their fair share of the national cake," and the "inmates" do not perceive any purpose in voting as they are deeply disenfranchised from their Ghanaian society, government, and regional or federal relief or assistance programs (Awaf 2015, 1).

Modern lawmakers, police, and members of the legal profession who have in the past attempted to regulate, investigate, and/or enforce litigation and/or criminal penalties for the unmerited prosecution of witches have been confounded and crushed under the weight of questionable testimonies, dubious circumstantial evidence, and random accusations. Historically, the cross-examination of such witchcraft trial testimonies find legal and police professionals hard-pressed to decipher between witnesses' factual (lucid consciousness), dream-state (sensory, cognitive, and emotional episodes during sleep), or purposely fictionalized (simulated, invented, or imagined) state of mind. For example, in Cameroon, Elias Bongmba uses the Limbum term "tʉ" to describe different activities that relate to witchcraft and argues that certain uses of "tʉ" are neutral. Scholars have drawn a sharp distinction between local methods of adjudication and the practice of modern jurisprudence (which has seen court litigation accusing others of using witchcraft against them). This has raised new questions about the possibilities and efficiency of any litigation of witchcraft accusations in constitutional courts. In the past, local justice systems and religious rituals were used as mechanism of accusing people as witches, yet these methods of adjudication were often restrained under the Colonial judicial system. In the last several decades the courts have been used by some individuals to press charges against suspected witches, while some states and human rights activists have argued that these court charges are not lawful or valid indictments as they violate the human rights of the accused (Fisiy 1990 and Aschroft 2015).

At the outset of this social enigma, it may also seem easy to point a critical finger at the local chiefs of the so-called witches' villages. Yet, with a more thorough grasp of the social intricacies, we see a local (usually via a familial linage) leader who has his/her proverbial 'hands tied' by deep-rooted beliefs in this systemic and supernatural system of justice. Gnani's (now deceased) former chief, Zachari Mahama, explained his role as such:

> When my people declare that a woman is a witch I have to send her away for her own protection. Otherwise she may be beaten to death. I am not happy to banish women but I am compelled to do so to keep the peace in my village. The tests are all done according to our faith so it would also be very hard for me to rule against the priests and defend someone they have found to be a witch. (Holland 2005, 62)

For whatever reasons—mental health issues, inequitable social power, revenge, erroneous advice, or a genuine certitude in their own traditional powers—some women have voluntarily confessed in courts of law that they are, indeed, guilty of witchcraft. One such self-confessed witch in 2009 in Harare, Zimbabwe, was sentenced under a 2006 law known as the Criminal Law Codification and Reform Act. This act demands "proof" that a person has supernatural powers and that they are using them to harm others (Vickers 2006, 1).

In Zimbabwe in 1899, colonial settlers made it a crime to accuse someone of being a witch or wizard—wary of the witch hunts in Europe a few centuries earlier that saw many people burned at the stake after such accusations. There are many other accounts of the use of magic, and the new law effectively legitimizes many practices of traditional healers. These include rolling bones to foretell the future, divination, attempts to communicate with the dead, using muti-traditional powders and fetishes—to ensure the desired sex of a child. But there will be some legal grey areas, like whether it is legal for a husband to place some charms in his bedroom—charms that may injure his wife if she is unfaithful. The Witchcraft Suppression Act was used fairly frequently, but prosecuting someone under the new legislation may prove problematic. The government acknowledges that supernatural powers exist—but prohibits the use of magic to cause someone harm.

Though estimates vary, as of 2015, an estimated 500 to over 1,000+ women and men and some 300 children are relegated to Ghana's witches' camps. In 2015, ActionAid was one of the agencies tasked with attempting to shut down all six camps, on the grounds that witchcraft accusation is now officially considered a form of human rights abuse. The ActionAid worker also added that the "conditions in the camps are so terrible. They don't have access to food, no access to even clean water. They don't have any income, they don't work" (Dunn 2015, 1).

Several international and national human rights agencies have attempted to address violence against condemned witches, including the 2002 U.N. Special Rappoteur on Violence Against Women, the 2009 U.N. Special Rappoteur on Extra-Judicial Killings, the U.N. High Commission on Refugees, UNICEF, the European Parliament (child witchcraft allegation policy briefing paper by Hanson and Ruggiero from 2013), as well as NGOs such as Save the Children, HelpAge International, Pan-African Organization for Research and Prevention of Violence against Women and Children, Stepping Stones, the Presbyterian church's Go-Home Project, and others (Ashforth 2015, and Tetzlaff 2015). More local grassroots efforts have been afforded via some of Ghana's own organizations, including the: Anti-Witchcraft Allegation Campaign Coalition (AWACC), Akrowa Aged-Life Foundation, Witch-Hunt Victims Empowerment Project, Ghanaian Aging Resources (GAR), Ghana Association of Persons Living with Albinism (GAPA), AfiKids, Pan African Organisation for Research and Protection of Violence on Women and Children (PAORP-VWC), Southern Sector Youth and Women's Empowerment Network, and others. Witchcraft accusation and persecution, also known as WAP, has become so global that the UNHCR and Fahamu Refugee Program offered a two-day course at Oxford University in 2010 for lawyers working on witchcraft asylum cases:

> Accusations of witchcraft are occurring today in communities around the globe. Startling accounts of torture, starvation, abandonment and death have been documented. Accused witches have been executed by hanging, burying alive, drowning and burning, with paraffin or petrol thrown at them to ignite the fire. Victims are often from vulnerable groups: the elderly, the disabled, and increasingly over the past two decades, children. (UNHCR and Fahamu Trust, 2010)

In fact, the UK-based NGO Witchcraft and Human Rights Information Network (WHIRN) has formed a network to promote "awareness and understanding of human rights violations that are committed around the world due to the belief in witchcraft" (2015, 1). According to WHIRN, approximately 865 people experienced violations of their human rights in 2013 alone "due to belief in witchcraft and other malevolent beliefs" (Ashforth 2015, 10). Witchcraft 'juju rituals' can also be used to elicit obedience from illiterate people and naïve children. One such case in 2012 reported that a Nigerian man recruited and raped young Nigerian orphan girls and forced them into prostitution by using the teenage girls' hair, nails, and blood to 'cast a spell' of submission, which (if broken) would cause the girls to be rendered infertile, go insane, and die (Peachey 2012). Conversely, the desperate women at these condemned witches' villages have been reported to resort to prostitution to support themselves, as women and young girls in "extreme circumstances" are often driven to use "transactional sex to get food, shelter or protection" (Holter 2015, 2).

Adam Ashforth argues a human-rights approach to any anti-witchcraft programs will have significant challenges as well:

> The human-rights approach to witchcraft accusations denies their validity and forecloses the possibility of a trial, fair or otherwise. While there is much to be said for a bracing rationalism in all aspects of life, evidence from Africa over the past couple of centuries shows no sign that witchcraft narratives lose their plausibility as a result of people being told that witches do not exist. (2015, 6)

We were pleasantly surprised that many of the residents were willing to think of the subject in a broader context. For example, we asked several of them in the interviews questions about political and legal approaches in different ways. We asked about what the government of Ghana has done. We also raised questions which called for them to comment on the legal instruments of the country, for instance the constitution and liberties it guarantees everyone in Ghana and what happens when cases of witchcraft go to court if they ever do in Ghana. The leader of the community in the Gnani village told us that she has heard that the constitution has banned so many outmoded cultural practices. She expressed frustration at the situation and asked why these practices continue if the laws of the land have banned them. She also stated that she thinks some things have changed because in the past, if someone were suspected of being a witch in Ghana, that person was beaten to death, and nothing happened to the ones who killed the alleged witch. At that point, Bongmba interjected and said that that was also the case in his region in Cameroon. Bongmba also reported that he knows of a case in his village when a woman, who had been exiled and told not to return to the village, came back to pick up some cloths, she was beaten by some of the villagers. Not many days after the incident, she died. Bongmba said he thought she might have died of injuries sustained from that beating, but he did not have the proof. Elizabeth reported that her sister had been accused of being a witch and was beaten to death.

We think that some of the women have talked about their situation for some time now and some of them are ready to take an activist posture regarding their situation in the village. Magdalene was an animated individual and spoke with a lot of gestures. During the interview it became clear why she was so animated. She had been accused three times of being a witch. For many people being accused once is a nightmare that they live with for their lifetime, but three times we thought was too much for one person. She was sent to the village against her will. But thankfully, from her perspective the priest in the village declared that she was not a witch. Traditional rites and sacrifices were offered and she returned home. But when another person died, she was accused again of being responsible for that death and she was sent back to the witches' village and told to stay for good. When we asked again if she was a witch, she laughed and said that she was unfortunate that the husbands she married died and because she survived, people thought she was the one who killed others. This was obviously a dilemma for her and other women who survive their spouses. When we asked what could be done, she surprised us by stating that she thinks that women should speak to the people who can influence the decision makers to take these conflicts seriously. Something should be done to help people understand that these disputes caused by suspicions that others are witches are not good for people and their villages. She did not know exactly what the political leaders can do, but she felt it was time to talk to them and ask them to do something about their plight in the village. At this point it seemed as we were all enjoying the conversation because she clearly was thinking about the issues carefully. When we asked if she and her friends could organize and vote only for leaders who will promise to do something about the plight of women in the many witches' villages in Northern Ghana, she responded that with help they can do that because women could not wait for the men to help them with these issues.

GO HOME: RESTORATION AND RECONCILIATION

Humanitarian aid workers who have worked in Gnani see little modification in the collective Ghanaian posture toward witchcraft accusations. "Only education will allow these women back into society," stated Gnani NGO worker and International Needs Ghana director Rev. Walter Pimpong, "If Cholera kills people in a village they must understand that the problem comes from a disease that can be treated. If crops fail they must look for a reason in the soil" (Holland 2005, 63). As for what the future may hold, Pimpong is afraid this change will take a prolonged period and "many more women will be condemned before then" (Holland 2005, 63).

Regrettably, death may be the only peaceful reconciliation with their families and communities that many of these elderly condemned "witches" can hope for and wait upon.

The nonprofit organization ActionAID Ghana, our source here, organized a forum for all the stake holders in Ghana in November 2001 and submitted a position which called for a clear road map for such a transition. Such a plan would create conditions where the women would feel safe in their communities and be able to support themselves economically. While one can applaud the government's stand that confining women to a witch's village is unjust and violates the rights of the women (with the long-term objective to close such communities), such processes should take into consideration the psychological resonance, security, and spiritual atmosphere that these villages have provided. This is consistent with many of the recommendations given by ActionAID Ghana.

"We have to do a lot of work with their communities so that they are able to return without being lynched or subjected to reaccusation, for example if a cow jumps over a fence and knocks down something. We are going to have to disabuse people's minds and that takes a long time," explained Adwoa Kwateng-Kluvitse, ActionAid's country director in Ghana (Whitaker 2012, 1). In Kwateng-Kluvitse's opinion, the change will take no less than 10 to 20 years (Whitaker 2012).

Since so much has been said by the Ghanaian government and international community about dismantling the "camps" we thought we should talk to the residents of the villages about their perspective on those calls for the government to close down the villages. Our interviews were structured in such a way that we could approach the question in different ways. Sometimes, we asked the resident if she missed her home, then followed up by asking if she would like to go back to her home, if asked to do so. Many said that they wanted to stay in the witches' village.

One question we posed to the residents was the role of religion in effecting reconciliation between individuals, the families, and community. During the conversations we avoided using technical terms like "reconciliation" and instead referred to a common idea like making peace and returning to live in harmony with others in the village. The residents all understood the idea and some said that they would consider that if there were the people in the village willing to make to peace. Almost all of them reminded us that they were the ones who were driven out of their homes and villages, and that they did not have a platform on which to engage in the practice of reconciliation and peace. They reminded us that in many cases not even their relatives came to visit them at the witches' village, and no religious leaders or elders from their precious homes came to visit them.

The case of Magdalene illustrates this very well. She lived in the town of Sangul, Ghana, which is approximately 40 miles outside of the witches' village. She was accused of being responsible for the death of her husband's grandmother. In some African communities that would be considered unusual because her husband's grandmother would not have been considered a close relative that she could "deploy" witchcraft powers over her. Nonetheless, she was accused of being responsible for the death of her husband's grandmother. She had nine children with her deceased husband, three boys and six girls. In her discussions with us, she was unsure of witchcraft's existence, but argued that if witchcraft is real, then it is bad because the people who have such powers can use it to kill others. Given her strong convictions that she was not responsible for the death of her husband's grandmother, we asked her if she would consider returning home to live with her children, extended family members, and fellow neighbors. She stated emphatically that she would not go back: "They sacked me from there." We then raised the question from a religious perspective, and asked if as a Christian she should consider forgiving those people who accused her and return to live in the village. She said: "I could forgive because I understand that the church tells me to forgive. But I have fears that if I forgive and go back, I cannot know what they will do, or what I will do."

When we asked Mariamu, a devout Muslim, if religion plays any role in her life, she responded affirmatively. She still prays and fasts as required by the Islamic faith. She also said her advice to any woman who is accused is that she should welcome it with faith (as she has) as Allah is the one who does everything and has omnipotent power to control the lives of innocent people, even if they are wrongly accused.

Overwhelmingly, the residents of the village believe that religious organizations care about them. In a discussion, some of the women pointed out that so far, most of the faith-based organizations that have come to their aid are Christian-based nonprofits. Nonetheless, they did not suppose that this showed that the Islamic-based faith (which has been in the area for a long time) supports witchcraft or wants them to continue to suffer. In their opinion, it was rather an issue of resources and that the Christian organizations were from "wealthier" Western countries. The organizations that were mentioned included World Mission Possible which has made eight medical visits to the village, Action AID, and the Lewis Foundation. They were emphatic though that Islamic organizations need to do something or else they are going to lose members, who now see what Christians are doing and think the Christians care more for them than their own religious communities. They pointed to the fact that two new churches have opened in the area, and a school has been opened to educate their children. What some researchers have noted is that Ghanaian witch camps "are products of institutionalized state of exception" but they do serve two-fold specific functions within the social order, namely: accusations are "securitizing acts" that keep the general populace "safe" as the "danger" (i.e., public threat, collective fears) is "fixated in the body of the accused," thus this "biopoliticisation" removes the threat from society, making her a "legitimate target of violence" (Macdonald 2012, 5) and reducing her to "*homo sacer*" or "bare life" (Agamben1995). The vulnerable groups of condemned witches studied in this research can be said to exist under the auspices of Giorgio Agamben's bare life or as "*homo sacer*"—someone who subsists or endures a life within a government's law, yet is an exile in it, as they do not exercise their rights to vote. The "*homo sacer*" concept of the sacred (or the excluded, doomed, or accursed) man is Agamben's interpretation is based on an ancient Roman law: a person who is banned, may be killed by anyone, yet cannot be sacrificed during a religious ritual (1995). The Italian philosopher's ethico-politico stance on the "bare life" of people who are in a suspended state of "inclusive exclusion" within a government's constraints can be summed up as: "the so-called sacred and inalienable rights of man prove to be completely unprotected at the very moment it is no longer possible to characterize them as rights of the citizens of a state." Much like the reanimation of people living in a state of suspended animation, Ghanaian politics must shake off the confusion and general aporias that characterizes witchcraft accusations, including the aporia of bare life in these villages like Gnani.

RECOMMENDATIONS

The rationale for designating the topic of this book as a "paradox" is straightforward: Even an innocuous query concerning the topic of witchcraft is enough to silence even the most modern, enlightened, and learned Ghanaian. The topic rarely arises in "decent company" as contemporary Ghanaians do not in polite conversation (and certainly not with *Obroni* or foreigners) chat about witchcraft, and that "to mention witchcraft [is] to admit an interest" (Drucker-Brown 1993, 533). Therefore it's a "lose-lose" Catch-22 proposition. To quote Margaret Heffernan's book *Willful Blindness: Why Ignore the Obvious at Our Peril*: "You cannot fix a problem that you refuse to acknowledge" (2011).

The witch camp is not the problem; witchcraft accusations are the main issue. The pervasive belief in Ghana that people can harm others through witchcraft is the elephant in the room that must be called out, not the safe places which alleged witches flee to.

"Reintegrated women keep coming back to the camps because they continue to be abused and molested in their communities" (Adae Npong 2014).

Yet perhaps, some progress is being made: A recent court case [in which the AWACC provided legal support] ruled in favor of a family banished from their home due to witchcraft allegations. The court compelled their chief to reinstate the family. . . . This kind of progress is now happening at the grassroots level where the UN has so far been ineffective.

Meanwhile, the number of outcasts seeking refuge seemingly continues to grow, due to nationally acknowledged, presupposed, and distributed witchcraft ideologies. Apart from Gnani, where a few older men reside (at last count, there were less than 10), the rest of the camps are all populated by outcast women and their children (Npong 2014). Although any exact number of residents is difficult to determine, the Anti-Witchcraft Allegation Campaign Coalition-Ghana reports there are 29,928 alleged witches in seven witches' camps and 13,287 children living with them, all in northern Ghana;

with almost 99.9 percent of the condemned witches constituting women and children (Laary 2015).

And as the time-worn proverb warns that "desperate diseases must have desperate remedies," so too must the affliction inflicted by witchcraft accusations find a constructive cure. Accordingly, the authors respectfully submit the following recommendations to facilitate an end to the current need of witches' villages in Ghana. These recommendations are in an abridged and simplified listing in order to streamline the reader's enumeration of the recommendations; the discourse, defense, justifications, and supporting evidence(s) can be found in research's associated topics and aforementioned chapters. The following list states, in no particular order, the top ten recommendations the authors make for both long- and short-term transformations concerning the alleviation of witchcraft accusations and decreasing the need for witches' villages:

(1) In our opinion, in order to "shut down" witchcraft allegations (as opposed to the current focus on "shutting down" witchcraft camps) the Ghanaian government should first focus its ambition and resources on *censoring the national media's fascination and (hence general public's) preoccupation with witchcraft*. Gerbner's "Cultivation Theory" studies show that media "cultivates heavy viewers' social reality," and TV influences people's perceptions of the world in that "TV is where people learn about their world and culture" (Schneider et al 2012, 147). Parents can do a lot to limit their children's exposure to witchcraft-laden media content by banning certain TV, social media, and radio programs, and studying non-violent conflict-resolution techniques with their children. Ghanaians can get their policy decision-makers to enforce 'non-witchcraft' media content via the new "Content Standards Regulation 2015" (LI 2224) passed by Parliament on December 9, 2015, that allows the National Media Commission to "establish and maintain standards in the distribution of content of public electronic communication and broadcasting services" so they may revoke licenses, administer fines and/or imprison violators (News Ghana, 2015). As an example, the most prominent recurring theme in Nollywood-produced films is "the power of witchcraft and its omnipresence in Africa societies" (WHRIN 2013, 8). The unmitigated censorship and restricted access to films that depict content encompassing witch hunts, albino *"muti"* murders/sacrifices, child witches, as well as other misogynistic "bullying" anti-witchcraft/dark *juju* topics should be enacted. Politicians cannot order these women to simply "go home" without adequate preparation and public dialogue. Their "home" could conceivably only lead to yet another displacement; any "home" should guarantee not only their well-being but their safety from abuse, ill-treatment, marginalization, and/or stigma.

(2) Secondly, NGOs and government officials can utilize *street theater, traditional drama, dance, comedy, and song*, to reach out to members of the

witches' village, and media to reach members of the Ghanaian population at large (militia, religious leaders, traditional healers, civil society organizations, etc.). As one example, a captivating play or popular dance can be used to patently explain that red eyes (often associated with witchcraft) can be caused by working over smoky cooking fires.

(3) As a third step, men and women should be trained as *paralegal advisers* to provide legal support, advice on land, inheritance, and marriage rights.

(4) Another recommendation we propose is for the anti-witchcraft accusation discourse in Ghana to take a more pronounced focus on these destructive indictments as a form of *elder abuse* rather than a focus on women's rights, gender-based violence, or an old woman's rights problem.

(5) Our fifth recommendation is more of a realization (or awareness) that intervention campaigns focused on replacing witchcraft (social issue) with medical sciences (explanatory framework) infrequently achieve success. Other intervention campaigns (that have attempted to influence HIV/AIDS and substance abuse) have uncovered that: *One moral (or scientific) system cannot simply replace another as an explanatory framework or means of resolving social drama* (Crampton 2013; Farmer 1990; Roy et al. 2011). So while Dr. Paul Farmer's medical work in Haiti with AIDS patients clearly noted that 'new' medical terms and diseases (as "explanatory models") may become known by the general populace—the "accompanying changes in medical rationality seldom seem to follow" (1990, 21). Farmer goes on to note that abuses of "cultural specificity" are "particularly insidious in discussions of suffering in general and of human rights abuses specifically," allowing cultural difference (on the verge of cultural determinism) to be used to "explain away assaults on dignity and suffering," in that culture "does not explain suffering; it may at worst furnish an alibi" (Farmer 1990, 48–49). One program was successful in fighting fallacious HIV/AIDs and "Virgin Cure" beliefs in Malawi by recruiting former traditional "cleansers" to revisit villages they previously served and condemning the tradition they once practiced as foolish, dangerous, and unwise (Radford 2013).

(6) Voting rights must not only be reestablished to exiled witches, but unimpeded voting access made possible through unrestricted transport modes, voter-education campaigns (specifically aimed at teaching semi-literate and illiterate residents), and open-access political assemblies and debate forums conducted in elementary-level language suited for the (primarily) poorly educated audience. Gnani's condemned witches not only suffer from the nation's economic neglect, but also a structural violence-based form of political repression. According to *The Economist*, research has shown that illiterate citizens are "less likely to cast a vote at all, and more likely to spoil their vote if they do," plus they are, "likely to be persuaded to sell their votes, or tricked or intimidated into voting for crooks and thugs" (2014, 1). According to the same article, voter-education campaigns, and face-to-face methods

that utilize picture guides, street theatre, and election-day simulations have proven successful in African countries in teaching illiterate citizens how to vote.

(7) There are incalculable direct and indirect local, regional, and national costs associated with witchcraft villages damaging Ghana's international human right record, including (but not limited to): a decrease in foreign-direct investments (FDI), damage to foreign companies' reputations (linking company to said violations), a volatile social instability (which can lead to political unrest and civil conflict), as well as a plethora of other issues. Nonetheless, to be more succinct, "studies suggest that human-rights violations, in fact, deter FDI [foreign-direct investments]" (Garriga and Phillips 2014). According to Lorenz Blume and Stefan Voigt's research published in "The Economic Effects of Human Rights": "Basic human rights have indeed a positive effect on investment," whereas, "Social rights, in turn, are not conducive to investment in physical capital but do contribute to productivity improvement" (2007, 538).

(8) Finally NGO partners and local communities must add healthcare infrastructures (clinics), improve camp sanitation facilities, and introduce community-driven farming solutions, such as Heifer International's programs—that build the capacity of vulnerable small-scale farmers, especially women, to secure their livelihoods in a sustainable scheme that creates self-reliance. The core of Heifer International's farming model is referred to by the U.S.A.-based NGO as "Passing on the Gift" where families share their training, and "pass on" the first female offspring of their (Heifer-donated goat/cow/chicken) original livestock to another impoverished local family, whereby the community's families become donors and proactive participants in developing their communities. Once the condemned witches in the villages see improvements in their health, mental health, and livelihoods, further community and gender-empowerment programs could follow suit.

(9) One efficacious antidote to witchcraft allegations involving sickness and death would be to educate the new generation of Ghana's young children on the medical and scientific knowledge encompassing human physiology. There is a great need to introduce public health education concepts to primary, middle-school, and high-school students, including (but not limited to): Human Anatomy and Physiology (explain neurological disorders like epilepsy), Substance-Abuse Prevention, Disease Prevention, HIV/AIDS Education, First Aid, CPR and Personal Safety, Mental Health, Injury and Violence Prevention, Basic Nutrition, Human Genetics (to explain albinism), Health and Fitness, Sexual Abuse Prevention, and Community Health.

(10) There must be some form of ethical and non-corrupt law enforcement and/or policing made available to these Northern Region citizens protect lives and livelihoods, defend civil liberties, and secure the safety of its fellow citizens. Only then perhaps can these residents begin to decrease these

witchcraft accusations used as mob-justice, vigilante, and self-policing social mechanisms. Additionally, Ghana must offer an unbiased and efficacious law enforcement, homicide detectives, criminal special investigation units (CSI), as well as government official(s) who would investigate any violent, sudden, or suspicious death (i.e., coroners, forensic scientists, toxicologists, pathologists) in order to verify the cause of death via empirical evidence. Law enforcement is one of the most noble and selfless occupations in society, however Ghanaian police are infamous for their alleged corruption and bribery. One of the first guidelines Flowers and Richter quickly learned was on no occasion to trust or rely on assistance from local police. On innumerable occasions, our vanloads of volunteer healthcare providers have been stopped by Ghanaian police (in every region) for preposterous and illegal citations such as: driving without a flashlight (during the day); driving without a fire extinguisher (not required); passport checks and control (after legal immigration entry); the transport of "many boxes"; and many other absurd excuses in order to elicit 2 to 10 cedis from us. According to the 2014 "Socio-economic and Governance Survey" conducted by the Institute of Economic Affairs reported that 23 percent of the 1,200 randomly sampled Ghanaians regard "nearly all policemen" as corrupt, with only 4.4 percent saying "not all" were corrupt (GBA 2015, 1). This report points to the widespread bribery and corruption, stating that the "most likely" bribes in the country stem from attempts to "avoid a problem with the police," or, "avoiding a fine or arrest" from police (GBA 2015, 1). The global corruption watchdog, Transparency International, ranked Ghana 61st out of 175 countries in its 2014 "Corruption Perception Index"—and rated Ghana Police Service as the most corrupt state institution in their 2013 "Global Corruption Barometer" (GBA 2015). So what should be deemed as an honorable police code of behavior? According to International Association of Chiefs of Police, the following "Law Enforcement Oath of Honor" is recommended as a representational statement of commitment to virtuous policing behavior:

> On my honor, I will never betray my badge, my integrity, my character, or the public trust. I will always have the courage to hold myself and others accountable for our actions. I will always uphold the constitution, my community, and the agency I serve. (International Association of Chiefs of Police 2015)

Additionally "enhancing integrity within an organization, leaders must ensure the oath is recited frequently and displayed throughout the organization as well as ensuring ethical mentoring and role modeling are consistent, frequent and visible" (International Association of Chiefs of Police 2015).

As Crampton notes in her article "No Peace in the House: Witchcraft Accusations as an 'Old Woman's Problem' in Ghana": "the reduction of witchcraft to a problem of violence against women of whatever age misses a larger social context of ambiguity, contingency, and negotiation," and that a solution to "banish beliefs" or coerce a social transformation does not "seem to be taking root in the country as a whole" (2013, 209).

WITCHES' VILLAGES ARE SYMPTOMS — NOT THE DISEASE

As we three co-authors were struggling between the conflicting micro- and macro-cosms of Western medicine, ancient sub-Saharan witchcraft, contemporary feminism, and Ghanaian tradition, I repeatedly found myself revisiting a favorite epitaph by renowned ethnobotanist, explorer, and scientist Wade Davis: "*The world in which you were born is just one model of reality. Other cultures are not failed attempts at being you; they are unique manifestations of the human spirit.*" Indeed, in this abridged quasi-ethnographic piece of biosocial research, we seek to furtively, albeit momentarily, remove our national "rose-colored glasses" and don those of another known—yet quite unknown—culture and people. And "therein lies the rub" of any and every people's existence, comparably and simultaneously both delightful and dreadful.

In 2014 Bonyase's small witches' camp was disbanded by the Ghanaian government to erase what it considers a stain on its human rights record. Shortly after this sanctuary was shut down, a local non-governmental organization, the Anti-Witchcraft Allegation Campaign Coalition (AWACC), wrote a letter to the Minister for Gender, Children and Social Protection drawing her attention to their position on this issue. It succinctly states:

> We do agree and support the idea to close these homes. However, we propose that the process be carried out through a long-term planning alongside various innovative interventions (looking at between 7 to15 years) with more focus on intensive public education, undertaking gradual processes, multi-partnership and consultations at all levels to avoid duplication of efforts, bearing in mind the interest of the victims, their families and communities these women will be re-integrated to eliminate backlash. (Laary 2015)

The group makes it clear that closing of the witches' camps has little or no bearing on the permanent resolution of issues of accusations and banishment. The AWACC added that: "It is sad and disappointing to note that, only three days after the ceremony held in Tamale (in December 2014) to have Bonyase officially closed, two out of the five outcast women had to immediately relocate to the Gnani home, near Yendi" (Laary 2015).

At the time of this book's publication, Ghana's Minister for Gender, Children and Social Protection, Nana Oye Lithur, announced future plans to shut down a second northern camp, the Gushiegu witches' camp—hence two mis-steps in an erroneous direction. These top-down machinations serve no purpose other than to further endanger these already-marginalized victims of accusation. Hence the witches' camp is not the problem—it is merely the *symptom*—not the core *disease*.

Much like "legislating" or "criminalizing" other social, moral, and/or religious norms and practices such as child brides, female genital cutting (also known as Female Genital Mutilation [FGM]), and widowhood rites—have historically proven rather ineffective. As one example, when FGM was legally banned in Senegal in 1999 the "threat of criminal sanctions is weighed against the effects of defying social norms, and this calculus is strongly influenced by the degree to which the cultural value has been called into question" (Shell-Duncan et al. 2014, 831). In Shell-Duncan et al.'s three years of research, two prevalent theories on social regulation were assessed: the law and economics, and the law and society paradigms—with divergent predictions to individual behavior that were affected by four factors: knowledge of the law; assessments on enforceability; use of formal legal system for resolution and/or recourse in the cases of disputes; and the ability of law to alter individual behavior (2014). The study revealed that legal coercion alone was insufficient as a singular change instrument. Although Rahman and Toubia notably argue that: "law can be a useful tool for change, giving NGOs and individuals greater leverage in persuading communities to abandon the practice" (2000, 13).

Incontrovertibly, the aforementioned details and data that point to the possibility of a "purely medical cause" of these people's illnesses or deaths calls into direct question the various traditions, suspicions, convictions, and uses of witchcraft allegations, and traditional authority leadership. The ubiquitous Ghanaian beliefs that others can cause physical, metaphysical, spiritual, and fiscal harm through witchcraft is the conspicuous elephant in Ghana's living room, so to speak—a brute so large and insufferable you simply cannot ignore it. Yet before the international realm of Westerners and Americans criticize or condemn Ghana for the 500 to 1,400 women that have been banished to witches' villages, one must also consider the thousands—perhaps tens of thousands—of people that the United States has incarcerated (and continues to hold) some would claim excessively, prejudicially (discriminatorily) and/or unjustly. The unadulterated fact is that in 2015 the United States comprises less than 5 percent of the world's population, yet imprisons approximately 25 percent of the world's total prison population (Lee 2015). Hence no currently functioning national government is above reproach.

In the end, "social transformation" legislation can serve to increase local awareness, and work most effectively when laws emerge from community demand, enjoy respectful, local "culturally mediated" grassroots support to uphold them, and are not resented in rural communities as a "criminalization of culture" (Shell-Duncan 2014, 831, and the Council on Foreign Relations 2016). Much like the reanimation of people living in a state of suspended

animation, Ghanaian politics must shake off the confusion and general aporias that characterizes witchcraft accusations, including the aporia of bare life
in these villages like Gnani. Indeed, Ghanaian "witch camps are born out of
and preserved by an institutionalized state of exception," and in order to
suspend the use of witches' villages, "the state of exception and existential
fears behind witch hunts must be addressed" (Tetzlaff 2015, 79).

Yet condemned witches' villages would not have emerged without the
previous advent of witch hunts. So no more than a pen can be blamed for
poor writing, or the mailman blamed for bringing mail bearing bad news—
witches' villages are byproducts, not geneses. In the United States, the cli-
chéd idiom we use is: Don't shoot the piano player! In other words, if the
piano is out of tune, the pianist playing isn't at fault; rather the piano's defect
must first (initially) be addressed before anyone can be expected to perform
well.

And the incidence of abuse towards older people, and women in particular, is predicted to increase as many countries are experiencing rapidly aging
populations, and many more women are outliving their (male) spouses. The
time is imminent for a more resolute institutional response for elderly wom-
en, who are (already) the most vulnerable globally to endure the hardships of
old age, poverty, widowhood, and a lack of a safe societal refuge.

In the end, exiling people to witches' villages is a non-durable non-
solution to a social conundrum. Ghana's witch camps endure as tangible
symptoms, if you will, and not the disease. Little benefit will come from a
few hastily applied political Band-Aids that merely focus on erasing the
nation's stained human rights record—without the unconditional eradication
of modern-day witchhunts that sanction the continued victimization of some
of society's most vulnerable members.

Appendix

Diopter Tolerances for Recycled Eyeglasses — WMP

Table 6.1. Diopter Tolerances for Recycled Eyeglasses—WMP

SPHERE (+) SINGLE VISION	CYLINDER TOLERANCE	RIGHT VS. LEFT LENS ALLOWANCE
+0.50 diopter	0	0.25 diopter
+0.75 to +1.00 diopter	0.25 diopter	0.25 diopter
+1.25 to 2.00 diopter	0.50 diopter	0.50 diopter
+2.00 and higher	0.75 diopter	0.75 diopter
SPHERE (-) SINGLE VISION	CYLINDER TOLERANCE	RIGHT VS. LEFT LENS ALLOWANCE
-0.50 diopter	0.25 diopter	0.25 diopter
-0.75 to -1.50 diopter	0.50 diopter	0.50 diopter
-1.75 to -3.50 diopter	0.75 diopter	1.00 diopter
* No inventory on progressives, multifocal (bifocal or trifocal) or eyeglasses below +/- 0.50 diopters	*on higher powers than listed above, the cylinder power can be raised by an additional 0.25 diopters	*on higher powers than listed above, the allowable difference can be raised by an additional 0.25 diopters
	*on powers higher than +/- 6.00 to +/- 8.00 diopters tolerances can be increased by an additional 0.25	*on powers higher than +/- 6.00 to +/- 8.00 diopters allowances can be increased by an additional 0.25

Bibliography

ActionAid. *Condemned without Trial: Women and Witchcraft in Ghana.* London: U.K., 2012.

Acolatse, Esther E. *For Freedom or Bondage: A Critique of African Pastoral Practices.* Grand Rapids: Eerdmans Publishing, 2014.

Adam, Hajia Amina. "What goes on at Gambaga 'witches' camp'"? *The Mirror.* August 5, 2000.

Adams, Patch. *Gesundheit!* Rochester: Healing Arts Press, 1993.

Adinkrah, Mensah. "Witchcraft Accusations and Female Homicide Victimization in Contemporary Ghana." *Violence against Women.* 2004 10(4): 325–356.

Adinkrah, Mensah. *Witchcraft, Witches, and Violence in Ghana.* New York: Berghahn, 2015.

Agamben, Giorgio. *Homo Sacer: Sovereign Power and Bare Life.* Connecticut: Stanford University Press, 1998.

Agyemang, Fred. *Accused in the Gold Coast.* Tema: Ghana Publishing Corporation, 1972.

Akrong, Abraham. Researching the Phenomenon of Witchcraft. *Journal of African Christian Thought.* 1999:(2) 44–46.

Akrong, Abraham. "A Phenomenology of Witchcraft in Ghana." In *Imaging Evil: Witchcraft Beliefs and Accusations in Contemporary Africa,* 53–66. Edited by Gerrie Ter Haar. Trenton, New Jersey: African World Press, 2007.

Akudugu, Mamudu A., and Mahama, Edward, S. "Promoting Community-Based Conflict Management and Resolution Mechanisms in the Bawku Traditional Area of Ghana." *Peace Research: The Canadian Journal of Peace and Conflict Studies.* 2011(43): 80–103.

Amoah, Elisabeth, "Women Witches and Social Change in Ghana." In *Speaking of Faith: Cross Cultural Perspectives on Women, Religion and Social Change,* 77–87. Edited by Diane Eckand Devaki. London: Women's Press, 1986.

Amnesty International. "Gambia: Hundreds Accused of Witchcraft and Poisoned in Government Campaign." *AllAfrica.com.* March 18, 2009. www.cnn.com/2009/WORLD/africa/03/18/gambia.amnesty.witchcraft (accessed September 20, 2015).

Amoah, Elizabeth. "Femaleness: Akan Concepts and Practices." In *Women, Religion and Sexuality: Impact of Religious Teachings on Women,* 129–153. Edited by Jeanne Becher. Geneva: World Council of Churches, 1990.

Ampofo, Oku. "The Traditional Concept of Disease, Health and Healing with the Christian when the Christian Church is Confronted." *The Ghana Bulletin of Theology* 1967(3.2):6–9.

Anderson, Benedict. *Imagined Communities: Reflections on the Origin and Spread of Nationalism.* London: Verso Press, 2006.

Apter, Andrew. "Atinga Revisited: Yoruba Witchcraft and the Cocoa Economy 1950–51." In *Modernity and Its Malcontent: Ritual and Power in Postcolonial Africa,* 111–128. Edited by Jean Comaroff and John Comaroff. Chicago: University of Chicago Press, 1993.

Ardener, E. "Witchcraft Economics and the Continuity of Belief." In *Witchcraft Accusations and Confessions*. Edited by Mary Douglas. London: Tavistock, 1970.

Asamohh-Gyadu, J. Kwabena. *African Charismatics: A Study of Independent Indigenous Pentecostalism in Ghana*. Leiden: Brill, 2005.

Asamoah-Gyadu, J. Kwabena. *Sighs and Signs of the Spirit Ghanaian Perspectives on Pentecostalism and Renewal in Africa*. Oxford: Regnum Books, 2015.

Asare Opoku, Kofi Asare. *West African Traditional Religion*. Accra: FEP International Private Ltd., 1978.

Ashforth, Adam. "Witchcraft, Justice, and Human Rights in Africa: Cases from Malawi." *African Studies Review* 2015(58): 5–38.

Ashforth, Adam. "Witchcraft, Violence, and Democracy in the New South Africa." *Cahiers d'Études Africaines* xxviii. 1998(2–4): 505–532.

Assimeng, Max. *Religion and Social Change in West Africa: An Introduction to the Sociology of Religion*. Accra: Ghana University Press, 1989.

Auslander, M. "Open the Wombs! The Symbolic Politics of Modern Ngoni Witchfinding." In *Modernity and its Malcontents: Ritual and Power in Postcolonial Africa*. Edited by J. Comaroff and J.L. Comaroff. Chicago: University of Chicago Press, 1993.

Awaf, Abdul-Karim Mohammed. "Witches Camps in Northern Ghana—Reality or an Illusion?" Accra: *Modern Ghana*, March 26, 2015.

Baëta, C. G. *Prophetism in Ghana: A Study of 'Spiritual Churches'*. London: SCM Press, 1962.

Bauman, Norman. "How to Use Evidence-Based Medicine in Wound Care." Presentation at Vascular and Endovascular Issues Techniques and Horizons (VEITH) Symposium 2007.

BBC News. "Ghanaian Director's Film 'The Cursed Ones' Tackles Issue of Witchcraft." London: *BBC News Focus on Africa*. November 3, 2015.

Bediako, Kwame. *Theology and Identity: The Impact of Culture upon Christian Thought in the Second Century and Modern Africa*. Oxford: Regnum Books, 1992.

Bever, Edward. Witchcraft Fears and Psychosocial Factors in Disease. *Journal of Interdisciplinary History* 2000 30(4): 577.

Bierlich, B. *The Problem of Money: African Agency and Western Medicine in Northern Ghana*. New York: Berghahn Books, 2007.

Blume, Lorenz and Stefan Voigt. "The Economic Effects of Human Rights." KYKLOS, 2007 60(4):509–538.

Boateng, Michael. "Albinos Banished From Atebubu." Accra: *Ghanaian Chronicle*, June 4, 2015.

Boissy, Raymond and James Nordlund. "Dermatologic Manifestations of Albinism." *Medscape*, Oct. 21, 2014. http://emedicine.medscape.com/article/1068184-overview (accessed on March 31, 2015).

Bongmba, Elias Kifon. *African Witchcraft and Otherness*. Albany: State University of New York Press, 2001.

Boulaga, Fabien E. *Christianity without Fetishes: An African Critique and Recapture of Christianity*. Maryknoll, New York: Orbis Books, 1981.

Boyer, Paul and Stephen Nisssembaum. *Salem Possessed: The Social Origins of Witchcraft*. Massachusetts: Harvard University Press, 1974.

Brugiavani, Agar and Noemi Pace. "Extending Health Insurance: Effects of the National Health Insurance in Ghana." *European Report on Development*. Aug. 2010.

Buvinić, Mayra, Medici, André, Fernández, Elisa, and Ana Cristina Torres. "Gender Differentials in Health." In *Disease Control Priorities in Developing Countries*. 2nd Ed. Edited by Jameson et al. World Bank, Geneva: The International Bank for Reconstruction and Development / The World Bank Group, 2006.

Caporael, Linnda. "Ergotism: The Satan loosed in Salem?" *Science* 1976 (192): 21–26.

CIA World Factbook. "Physician Density: France, Ghana, and United States." Washington, D.C.: Central Intelligence Agency. http: www.cia.gov/library/publications/the-world-factbook/geos/gh.html (accessed Feb. 20, 2016).

Ciekawy, Diane. "Policing Religious Practice in Contemporary Coastal Kenya." *Political and Legal Anthropological Review*. May 1997.

Ciekawy, Diane. "Utsai as Ethical Discourse: A Critique of Power from Mikikenda in Coastal Kenya." In *Dialogues of Witchcraft: Anthropological and Philosophical Exchanges.* Edited by Bond, George, and Diane Ciekawy. Athens: Ohio Press, 2001.

Cochrane, Kira. "Sick Cities: Why Urban Life is Breeding New illness Fears." *The Guardian.* Feb. 24, 2014.

Council on Foreign Relations. "Female Genital Cutting and the Law: Why Criminalization Isn't Enough." New York: *Council on Foreign Relations.* Feb. 2016.

Crampton, Alexandra. "No Peace in the House: Witchcraft Accusations as an 'Old Woman's Problem' in Ghana." *Anthropology & Aging Quarterly* 2013 2(34): 199–212.

Crane, Tim and Sarah Patterson (eds.) *History of the Mind–Body Problem.* New York: Routledge, 2000.

Crick, Malcolm. "Recasting Witchcraft." In *Witchcraft and Sorcery: Selected Readings.* Edited by M. Marwick. London: Penguin Books, 1970.

Damasane, Paul. "The Gender Element in Witchcraft in Zimbabwe." *Sunday News*, Nov. 3, 2009.

Daswani, G. "Transformation and Migration among Members in a Pentecostal Church in Ghana and London." *Journal of Religion in Africa* 2010 40(4):442–474.

Debrunner, Hans. *Witchcraft in Ghana: A study on the Belief in Destructive Witches and its Effects on the Akan Tribes.* Accra, Ghana: Presbyterian Book Depot, 1961.

Development News Africa. "GHANA: Report Reveals That Witchcraft, FGM And Widowhood Rites as the Most Harmful Traditional Customs in Northern Ghana." *Development News Africa.* Nov. 4, 2015.

Dobson, Mary. *Disease: The Extraordinary Stories behind History's Deadliest Killers.* United Kingdom: Quercus, 2007.

Dophyne, Florence Abena. *The Emancipation of Women: An African Perspective.* Accra: Ghana Universities Press, 1991.

Douglas, Mary, ed. *Witchcraft Confessions and Accusations.* London: Tavistock, 1970.

Doucet, A. and N. S. Mauthner. "Feminist methodologies and Epistemology." In *Handbook of 21st Century Sociology*, 36–42. Edited by B. Clifton and D. Peck. Thousand Oaks Press, California: Sage, 2006.

Dovlo, Elom. "Witchcraft in Contemporary Ghana." In *Imaging Evil: Witchcraft Beliefs and Accusations in Contemporary Africa*, 67–92. Edited by Terrie Ter Haar. New Jersey: Africa World Press, 2007.

Drucker-Brown, S. "Mamprusi Witchcraft, Subversion, and Changing Gender Relations." London: *Africa* 1993 63(4): 531–549.

Dugbartey, Anthony, and Kofi Bobi Barimah. "Public Health: Traditional Beliefs and Knowledge Base about Epilepsy among University Students in Ghana." *Ethnicity and Disease* 2013 23:1–5.

Dunaway, David, and Ian Berger. "Worldwide Distribution of Visual Refractive Errors." Presentation to the International Society for Geographic and Epidemiologic Ophthalmology. InFOCUS Center for Primary Eye Care Development, University of Houston, 1998.

Dunn, Carolyn. "Ghana Witch Camps Shutting Down, Leaving Accused in Limbo." *CBC News,* March 7, 2015.

Economist, The. "Illiterate Voters: Making their Mark." Mumbai: *The Economist*, April 5, 2014.

Evans-Pritchard, Edward E. *Witchcraft, Oracles, and Magic among the Azande.* London: Oxford University Press, 1937.

Fadiman, Anne. *The Spirit Catches You and You Fall Down: A Hmong Child, Her American Doctors, and the Collision of Two Cultures.* New York: Farrar, Straus and Giroux, 1997.

Farmer, Paul. "Sending Sickness: Sorcery, Politics and Changing Concepts of AIDS in Rural Haiti," *Medical Anthropology Quarterly*, 1990 4(1): 6–27.

Farmer, Paul. *Infections and Inequalities: The Modern Plagues.* Los Angeles, California: University of California Press, 1999.

Farmer, Paul. *Pathologies of Power: Health, Human Rights, and the New War on the Poor.* Berkeley: University of California Press, 2005.

Field, Margaret. "Some New Shrines of the Gold Coast and their Significance." *Africa* 1940: 138–49.

Field, Margaret. *Religion and Medicine of the Ga People.* London: Oxford University Press, 1937.

Field, Margaret. *Search for Security: An Ethno-Psychiatric Study of Rural Ghana.* London: Faber & Faber, 1960.

Fisiy, C.F. "Palm Tree Justice in Bertua Court of Appeal: The Ordinary and the Witchcraft Cases." *Proceedings of the African Studies Center.* Leiden: African Studies Center, 1990.

Fisiy, C.F. and M. Rawlands. "Sorcery and the Law in Modern Cameroon." *Culture and History.* Neuchâtel, Switzerland: Bibliothèques de l'Université 1989: 63–84.

Flint, Karen Elizabeth. *Healing Traditions: African Medicine, Cultural Exchange, and Competition in South Africa.* Athens: Ohio University Press, 2009.

Fortes, M. and G. Dieterlen, eds. *African Systems of Thought.* London: Oxford University Press, 1965.

Fortes, Meyer. *Religion, Morality and the Person: Essays on Tallensi Religion.* Cambridge: Cambridge University Press, 1987.

Fortes, Meyer. *The Web of Kinship among the Tallensi.* London: Oxford University Press, 1949.

Galtung, Johan. "Kulturelle Gewalt." *Der Burger im Staat.* 1993 (43): 106.

Garriga Ana Carolina, and Brian Phillips "Foreign Aid as a Signal to Investors: Predicting FDI in Post-conflict Countries." *Journal of Conflict Resolution* 2014 58(2): 280–306.

Geert, Tom and Mark Manary. "75 Years of Kwashiorkor in Africa." *Malawi Medical Journal* 2009 21(3): 96–100.

Geschiere, Peter. *The Modernity of Witchcraft: Politics and the Occult in Postcolonial Africa.* Charlottesville: University of Virginia Press, 1997.

Ghana Broadcasting Association (GBA). "IEA survey Cites Ghana Police Service as Most Corrupt state institution." Accra: Ghana Broadcasting Association services. Feb. 26, 2015. http://gbcghana.com/1.2010459 (accessed Feb. 22, 2016).

Ghana Educational Services (GES). "Cultural Studies for Junior Secondary Schools." Accra: Ghana Ministry of Education and Culture. 1988: 137–138.

Ghana Health Service. "National Malaria Control Programme." Accra: 2009. http://www.ghanahealthservice.org/ghs-subcategory.php?cid=4&scid=41 (accessed Feb. 26, 206).

Ghana News Agency. "Survey Says Tuberculosis Prevalence in Ghana is High." Accra: *Ghana News Agency.* March 26, 2015.

Gifford, Paul. *African Christianity: Its Public Role.* Bloomington: Indiana University Press, 1998.

Gifford, Paul. *Ghana's New Christianity: Pentecostalism in a Globalising African Economy.* Bloomington: Indiana University Press, 2004.

Gilligan, James. "Violence: Reflections on a National Epidemic." *Vintage,* 1996.

Gray, Natascha. "Independent Spirits: The Politics of Policing Anti-Witchcraft Movements in Colonial Ghana 1908–1927." *Journal of Religion in Africa,* 35.2 (2005): 139–158.

Greaves, Mel. "Was Skin Cancer a Selective Force for Black Pigmentation in Early Hominin Evolution?" *Proceedings of the Royal Society,* February 26, 2014.

Green, Edward C. *Indigenous Theories of Contagious Disease.* Rowman & Littlefield Publishers, 1999.

Groenhout, Ruth. "The Brain Drain Problem: Migrating Medical Professionals and Global Health Care." *International Journal Feminist Approaches to Bioethics* 5(1):1–24.

Gyekye, Kwame. *Tradition and Modernity: Philosophical Reflections on the African Experience.* New York: Oxford University Press, 1997.

Haar, ter Gerrie, ed. *Imagining evil: Witchcraft beliefs and accusations in contemporary Africa.* Africa World Press Inc., 2007.

Hagan, George P. "Divinity and Experience: The Trance and Christianity in Southern Ghana." In *Vernacular Christianity: Essay in the social anthropology of religions.* Edited by Wendy James and Douglas H. Johnson. Oxford: JASO, 1988.

Harding, Sarah. "Rethinking Standpoint Epistemology: What is Strong Objectivity?" In *Feminist Epistemologies.* Edited by L. Alcoff and E. Potter. London: Routledge, 1993.

Heffernan, Margaret. *Willful Blindness: Why Ignore the Obvious at Our Peril.* Toronto: Doubleday Canada, 2011.

HelpAge USA. "Fighting Witchcraft Allegations." HelpAge USA, Kansas City: USA. http://www.helpage.org/helpageusa/what-we-do/older-women/older-womens-rights/fighting-witchcraft-accusations (accessed Jan. 5, 2016).

Holland, Heidi. *African Magic.* Johannesburg: Penguin Books 2005.

Hollenweger, Walter, J. *Pentecostalism: Origins and Developments Worldwide.* Massachusetts: Hendrickson Publishers, 2005.

Holter, Lauren. "The Disturbing Ways Women's Reproductive & Sexual Rights are Jeopardized During Crises." New York: *Bustle.* Dec. 3, 2015.

Hunt, Nancy Rose. *Suturing New Medical Histories of Africa.* Berlin: Lit Verlag 2013.

International Association of Chiefs of Police. "Law Enforcement Oath of Honor." International Association of Chiefs of Police. Alexandria, Virginia: http://www.iacp.org/What-is-the-Law-Enforcement-Oath-of-Honor (accessed Feb. 22, 2016).

Kgatla, S. T., Gerrie ter Haar, eds. *Crossing witchcraft barriers in South Africa. Exploring witchcraft accusations: Causes and solutions.* Netherlands: Utrecht University, 203.

Kirby, J.P. "Ghana Witches: Scratch Where it Itches!" *Mission & Culture,* 2012: 189–223.

Koram, Albin. "Witches' Camp: Cruelty against Women." *Weekly Spectator,* 20 September, 1997.

Kwatra, Anjali. "Condemned without Trial: Women and Witchcraft in Ghana." London: ActionAID, 2012. http://www.actionaid.org.uk/sites/default/files/doc_lib/ghana_report_single_pages .pdf (accessed September 7, 2015).

Laary, Dasmani. "Ghana: Freed Witches Relocate to Neighbouring Camps." *The Africa Report* Feb. 19, 2015.

Labuschagne, Gerard. "Features and Investigative Implications of *muti* Murder in South Africa." *Journal of Investigative Psychology and Offender Profiling* 2004 1(3): 191–206.

Lange, Maggie. "Witch Accusations Are a Real Problem in Ghana." *The Cut*, Oct. 22, 2013.

Larbi, Emmanuel Kingsley. *Pentecostalism: The Eddies of Ghanaian Christainity.* Accra: Center for Pentecostal and Charismatic Studies, 2001.

Lassey, A.T., Lassey , P.D., M. Boamah, "Career Destinations of University of Ghana Medical School Graduates of Various Year Groups." *Ghana Medical Journal* 1993, 47(2): 87–91.

Layhew, Ashley. "The Devil's in the Details: A Comprehensive Look at the Salem Witch Mania of 1692." *Journal of Student Historical Research.* Nashville: Tennessee State University, 2013.

Lee, Michelle. "Does the United States Really Have 5 Percent of the World's Population and One Quarter of the World's Prisoners?" *Washington Post.* April 30, 2015.

Lennon, K. & Whitford, M. (eds). *Knowing the Difference: Feminist Perspectives in Epistemology.* London, U.K.: Routledge, 2006.

Lowenstein, Daniel. "Approach to the Patient with Neurologic Disease." In *Harrison's Principles of Internal Medicine.* Edited by Longo, D. et. al. 18th ed. McGraw-Hill Professional, 2011.

Lwanga, Francis, Kirunda, Barbara, and Christopher Orach. "Intestinal Helminth Infections and Nutritional Status of Children Attending Primary Schools in Wakiso District, Central Uganda." *International Journal of Environmental Research and Public Health* 2012, 9: 2910–2921.

Lyons, Diane. "Witchcraft, Gender, Power, and Intimate Relations in Mura Compounds in Déla, Northern Cameroon." *World Archeology* 1998, 29(3)344–362.

Macdonald, Arnskov Connie. "Camping with Witches: Witch Hunts as Practices of Securitisation and Biopoliticisation." University of Copenhagen dissertation. Nov. 2012.

MacGaffey, Wyatt. "Death of a King, Death of a Kingdom? Social Pluralism and Succession to High Office in Dagbon, Northern Ghana." *Journal of Modern African Studies,* 2006, 44(1): 79–99.

Marx, John, Hockberger, Robert, and Ron Walls. *Rosen's Emergency Medicine: Concepts and Clinical Practice.* 8th Ed. Saunders, 2013.

Marx, Karl. *Hegel's Philosophy of Right (Zur Kritik der Hegelschen Rechtsphilosophie).* Edited by Joseph O'Malley. Cambridge University Press, 1970.

Matossian, MK. "Ergot and the Salem Witchcraft Affair." *American Science* 1982, 70(4): 355–357.

Mayo Clinic. "Stress and High Blood Pressure: What's the Connection?" Minnesota: Mayo Foundation for Medical Education and Research. http://www.mayoclinic.org/diseases-conditions/high-blood-pressure/in-depth/stress-and-high-blood-pressure/art-20044190 (accessed Feb. 20, 2016).

Mburu, John. "Witchcraft among the Wimbum." B.A. thesis in Philosophy, Regional Major Seminary, Bambui, Cameroon, 1979.

McLeod, Malcolm. "On the Spread of Anti-Witchcraft Cults in Modern Asante." In *Changing Social Structure in Ghana: Essays in the Comparative Sociology of a New State and an Old Tradition.* Edited by Jack Goody. London: International African Institute, 1975.

Meintjes, Sheila, Pillay, Anu, and Meredeth Turshen. *The Aftermath: Women in Post-Conflict Transformation.* London: Zed Books, 2001.

Merriam-Webster's Collegiate Dictionary. "Caligynephobia" and "Venustraphobia." Springfield, MA: Merriam-Webster Incorporated, 2015.

Meyer, Birgit. *Sensational Movies—Video, Vision and Christianity in Ghana.* Berkley: University of California Press, 2015.

Meyer, Birgit and Peter Pels, eds. *Magic and Modernity: Interfaces of Revelation and Concealment.* Stanford University Press, 2003.

Meyer, Birgit. *Translating the Devil: Religion and Modernity among the Ewe in Ghana.* Edinburgh: Edinburgh University Press, 1999.

Nabla, Moses. *Rehabilitation of the Witches in Gambaga- The Role of the Presbyterian Church of Ghana.* BA Hon. diss., University of Ghana, 1997.

News Ghana. "Ghana Adopts LI To Regulate Media Content: Ghana's Parliament has adopted an LI to Regulate the Content of Electronic Communication and Broadcasting Services." New Ghana, Accra: Dec. 14, 2015. http://www.newsghana.com.gh/ghana-adopts-li-to-regulate-media-content (accessed Feb. 22, 2016).

Nkatazo, Lebo. "Zimbabwe Outlaws Practise of Witchcraft." *New Zimbabwe,* April 24, 2006.

Nkatazo, Lebo. "Suspended Jail Term for Witch." *New Zimbabwe,* June 4, 2009.

Npong, Francis. "Witch Camps of Ghana." *Bust,* June/July 2014.

Nukunya, G.K. *Tradition and Change in Ghana: An Introduction to Sociology.* Accra, Ghana: GUP, 1992.

Oduyoye, Mercy Amba. *Daughters of Anowa: African Women & Patriarchy.* Maryknoll, NY.: Orbis Books, 1995.

Office of the United Nations High Commissioner for Human Rights (OHCHR). "Independent Expert on the Enjoyment of Human Rights by Persons with Albinism." Office of the United Nations High Commissioner for Human Rights.http://www.ohchr.org/EN/Issues/Albinism/Pages/IEAlbinism.aspx (accessed Dec. 13, 2015).

Office of the United Nations High Commissioner for Human Rights (OHCHR). "Mandate of the Independent Expert." Office of the United Nations High Commissioner for Human Rights. http://www.ohchr.org/EN/Issues/Albinism/Pages/Mandate.aspx (accessed Dec. 13, 2015).

Office of the United Nations High Commissioner for Human Rights (OHCHR). "Witchcraft in a Modern Age: Broken Communities and Recalcitrant Stigma." Office of the United Nations High Commissioner for Human Rights, Dec. 10, 2015. http://www.ohchr.org/EN/News-Events/Pages/WitchcraftInAModernAge.aspx (accessed Dec. 13, 2015).

Onyinah, Opoku. *Pentecostal Exorcism: Witchcraft and Demonology in Ghana.* Corset, United Kingdom: Deo Publishing, 2012.

Opoku, Kofi Asare. *West African Traditional Religion.* Accra, Ghana: FEP International Private Ltd, 1978.

Oppong, C. *Growing up in Dagbon.* Accra: Ghana Publishing Company, 1973.

Osam, Efua Idan. "Health Facilities Defy GHS Directive on NHIS." Accra: Citi News. http://citifmonline.com/2015/03/27/health-facilities-defy-ghs-directive-on-nhis (accessed Feb. 21, 2016).

Otto, Caitlin, and Shelley Haydel. "Exchangeable Ions Are Responsible for the In-Vitro Anti-bacterial Properties of Natural Clay Mixtures." Public Library of Science, *PLOS One.* 10 (1371): May 17, 2013.

Palmer, Karen. *Spellbound: Inside West Africa's Witch Camps.* New York: Free Press, 2010.

Papier, Keren, Williams, Gail, and Ruby Luceres-Catubig, et al. "Childhood Malnutrition and Parasitic Helminth Interactions." *Clinical Infectious Diseases* 59 (2014): 234–244.

Parish, Jane, "Chasing Celebrity: Akan Witchcraft and New York City" Ethnos, Vol. 78:2; 2013: 280–300.

Parish, Jane, "Circumventing Uncertainty in the Moral Economy: West African Shrines in Europe, Witchcraft and Secret Gambling" African Diaspora, 3 (2010): 77–93.

Peachey, Paul. "Man used Witchcraft to Traffic Children for Prostitution." *The Independent UK*, Sept. 7, 2012.

Pels, Peter. "The Magic of Africa: Reflections on a Western Commonplace," *African Studies Review* 41, 3 (1998): 193–209.

Pobeia, Bajin. "Triplets, a Taboo in some Lawra Communities." Wa: *Ghana News Agency.* April 26, 2011.

Pool, Robert. "There Must have Been Something: Interpretations of Illness and Misfortune in a Cameroonian Village." Ph.D. diss., University of Amsterdam, 1989.

Porter, Roy. *The Greatest Benefit to Mankind: A Medical History of Humanity.* New York: Norton and Company, 1997.

Pruett, Tom. Interview by Richter, Roxane. Personal Interview. Houston. Feb. 13, 2016.

Radford, Benjamin. "How Belief in Magic Spreads AIDS in Africa." *Discovery News*, March 21, 2013.

Radford, Benjamin. "Albino Toddler in Africa Killed for Witchcraft." *Discovery News,* March 2, 2015.

Rahman, Anika and Toubia, Rahid. *Female Genital Mutilation: A Guide to Laws and Policies Worldwide.* London: Zed Books, 2000.

Republic of Ghana. "Ghana's Chieftaincy Act of 2008." Accra: Government of the Republic of Ghana, June 16, 2008.

Republic of Ghana. "Constitution of the Republic of Ghana." Accra: Government of the Republic of Ghana, April 28, 1992.

Richter, Roxane. *Medical Outcasts: Gendered and Institutionalized Xenophobia in Undocumented Forced Migrants' Emergency Health Care.* Maryland: Rowman & Littlefield, 2015.

Roberts, Jani Farrell. "The Seven Days of My Creation: Tales of Magic, Sex and Gender," Bloomington, IL: iUniverse, 2002.

Rodlach, Alexander. *Witches, Westerners, and HIV: AIDS & Cultures of Blame in Africa* Left Coast Press, 2006.

Sackett, D., Rosenberg, W., Gray J., Haynes R, and W. Richardson. "Evidence-Based Medicine: What It Is and What It Isn't." *British Medical Journal* 1996 (312): 71–72.

Schneider, F., Gruman, J. and Coutts, L. (Eds.). *Applied Social Psychology: Understanding and Addressing Social and Practical Problems* (2nd ed.). Thousands Oaks, CA: Sage Publications, 2012.

Shell-Duncan, Bettina, Wander, Katherine, Hernlund, Ylva, and Amadau Moreau. "Legislating Change? Responses to Criminalizing Female Genital Cutting in Senegal." *Law and Society Review* 2013: 803–835.

Shinnie, P.L. and P.C. Ozanne. "Excavations at Yendi Dabari," *Transactions of the Historical Society of Ghana* 1962 (6): 87–118.

Schmoll, Pamela. "Black Stomachs, Beautiful Stones: Soul Eating Among Hausa in Niger," in *Modernity and its Malcontents: Ritual and Power in Postcolonial Africa,* edited by Jean and John Comaroff, 193–220. Chicago: University of Chicago Press, 1993.

Schnoebelen, Jill. "Witchcraft allegations, Refugee Protection and Human Rights: A Review of the Evidence," *New Issues in Refugee Research.* United Nations High Commission for Refugees. January (no. 169): 2009.

Shaw, Rosalind. Gender and the Structuring of Reality in Temne Divination: An Interactive Study. *Africa: Journal of the International African Institute* 55(1985): 286–303.

Southern Sector Youth and Women's Empowerment Network (SOSYWEN). *The Wasted Years: The Reality of the Witches Camps*. Accra, Ghana: Konsept Design, 2011.

South Africa Today. "African '*Muti*' Murders," *South Africa Today*, April 15, 2014.

Spanos, Nicholas P. and Gottlieb, Jack. "Ergotism and the Salem Village Witch Trials." *Science*. December 1976: 1390–1394.

Starkey, Marion. *The Devil in Massachusetts: A Modern Enquiry into the Salem Witch Trials*. New York: Doubleday Press, 1969.

Strochlic, Nina. "Africa's 'Albino Island,' " *The Daily Beast*, Feb. 19, 2015.

Tait, David. "Konkomba Sorcery," *Journal of the Royal Anthropological Institute of Great Britain and Ireland*. Jan-Dec 1954 (84):66–74.

Tait, David. "A Sorcery Hunt in Dagomba," *Africa: Journal of the International African Institute*. 1963 33(2):136–147.

Tau, Menes. "Albinism and whiteness—The origin of the Caucasian," *Grandmother Africa*, Nov 14, 2014.

Ter Haar, Gerrie. *Imagining Evil: Witchcraft Beliefs and Accusations in Contemporary Africa*. Trenton, New Jersey: Africa World Press, 2007.

Tetzlaff, Monica. "Alleged Witches Camps, Outcast Homes or Pwaanyankura-Foango," Indiana University South Bend: *IU International*. Oct. 24, 2015.

Twumasi, Patrick. "A History of Pluralistic Medical Systems: A Sociological Analysis of the Ghanaian Case." *Issue: A Journal of Opinion* 9:3, 29–34 Autumn 1979.

Twumasi, Patrick. *Medical Systems in Ghana: A Study in Medical Sociology*. Accra: Ghana Publishing Corporation, 1975.

United Nations. "U.N. findings flag violence, abuse of older women accused of witchcraft," UN Department of Economic and Social Affairs (UN DESA), June 2014. http://www.un.org/apps/news/story.asp?NewsID=48055#.Vox2LZVIiM8 (accessed on Jan 5, 2016).

United Nations Human Rights—Office of the High Commissioner. "International Covenant on Civil and Political Rights." Adopted and opened for signature, ratification and accession by General Assembly resolution 2200A (XXI) of 16 December 1966 entry into force 23 March 1976, in accordance with Article 49.

U.S. Department of State. "Human Rights Report for 2011: Ghana." Washington D.C.: U.S. Department of State, 2011. http://www.state.gov/j/drl/rls/hrrpt/2011humanrightsreport/index.htm (accessed on Feb. 14, 2016).

U.S. Department of State. "Human Rights Report for 2014: Ghana." Washington D.C.: U.S. Department of State, 2014. http://www.state.gov/j/drl/rls/hrrpt/humanrightsreport/index.htm (accessed on Feb. 14, 2016).

van der Geest, Sjaak. "From Wisdom to Witchcraft: Ambivalence towards Old Age in Rural Ghana." *Africa: Journal of the International African Institute*. 2002 72(3): 437–463.

Vickers, Steve. "Witchcraft Ban Ends in Zimbabwe." Harare: BBC. 2 July 2006.

Vision for Tomorrow Foundation. "Albinism's Impact on Vision." Illinois: Vision for Tomorrow Foundation. http://www.visionfortomorrow.org/albinisms-impact-on-vision (accessed Dec. 15, 2015).

West African Centre for International Parasite Control (WACIPC). "Project Document." Accra: Noguchi Memorial Institute for Medical Research, College of Health Sciences, University of Ghana. 2003. http://www.noguchimedres.org/wacipac/pdf/Project-doc.pdf (accessed Feb. 27, 2016).

Whitaker, Kati. "Ghana Witch Camps: Widows' Lives in Exile." *BBC News*, September 1, 2012.

Witchcraft & Human Rights Information Network (WHRIN). "Exploring the Role of Nollywood in the *Muti* Murders of Persons with Albinism." Lancashire, United Kingdom: WHRIN, Aug. 16, 2013.

Wilks, Ivor. "A Note on the Early Spread of Islam in Dagomba." *Transactions of the Historical Society of Ghana*. 1965(8): 87–98.

Wolf, Sebastian. *Ocular Fundus: From Findings to Diagnosis*. Thieme Medical Publishers, 2005.

World Health Organization (WHO) "Wealth, Health and Health Expenditure." NHA Policy Highlight. No. 4, 2010.

World Health Organization (WHO) "Health Financing in Ghana." World Health Organization Report for Ministerial Meeting of Health and Finance. Tunis, Tunisia. July, 2012.

Wolf, Sebastian. *Occular Fundus: From Findings to Diagnosis*. Thieme Medical Publishers, 2005.

Xaba, Thokozani. *Witchcraft, Sorcery or Medical Practice?* LAP Lambert Publications, 2010.

Yamoah, Michael. "The New Wave in Ghana's Film Industry: Exploring the Kumawood Model." *International Journal of ICT and Management* II (October 2014)2: 155–161.

Zakari, Alidu. Interview by Richter, Roxane. Personal interview. Gnani. Nov. 8, 2015.

Zimon, Henryk. "The Sacredness of the Earth among the Konkomba of Northern Ghana." *ANTHROPOS* 98 (2003): 421–443.

Index

About the Authors

Roxane Richter, Ph.D., E.M.T., is a current 2016–2017 Fulbright-Fogarty Fellow in Public Health, Sub-Saharan Africa (Ghana) researching prehospital trauma care in mass casualty motor-vehicle incidents and disasters. As an Emergency Medical Technician (EMT), Roxane's 16 years of frontline experience in international disaster aid and EMS have provided both the catalyst and forum for her to research global and gender healthcare disparities. She has authored *Medical Outcasts: Gendered and Institutionalized Xenophobia in Undocumented Forced Migrants' Emergency Health Care* (2015); "Disparity in Disasters: A Frontline View of Gender-Based Inequities in Emergency Aid and Healthcare" in *Anthropology at the Front Lines of Gender-Based Violence* (2011), and others. She has lectured at the World Congress on Emergency Medicine and Disasters, U.N. Association, Amnesty International, and more. Roxane serves as president of World Missions Possible, a nonprofit providing eye care, medical aid, and EMS capacity-building to 16 nations. She has traveled to 67 nations, serving with American Red Cross' Disaster Health Services and other nonprofits, providing free medical care to impoverished and disaster-stricken areas.

Thomas Flowers, D.O., has been practicing as an American Board of Emergency Medicine (ABEM)-certified physician since 1992. Dr. Flowers holds a B.S. in General Science from Oregon State University, and a Doctor of Osteopathy degree from ATSU/Kirksville College of Osteopathic Medicine. He spent a total 10 years on active duty in the U.S. Air Force, including three years in Great Britain. In 2006, Dr. Flowers became Medical Director of the Houston-based World Missions Possible, a nonprofit providing eye care, medical aid, and EMS capacity-building to 16 nations. Since then, he has led seven medical outreaches to rural Ghana from 2006 to 2016, as well as outreaches to South Africa, Swaziland, Zambia, and several homeless/indigent clinics in Houston and New Orleans. He has co-published two articles in peer-reviewed journals: "Gender-Aware Disaster Care: Issues and Interventions in Supplies, Services, Triage, and Treatment" in the *International Journal of Mass Emergencies & Disasters*, and "Gendered Dimensions of Disaster Care: Critical Distinctions in Female Psychosocial Needs, Triage, Pain Assessment, and Care" in the *American Journal of Disaster Medicine*.

Elias Kifon Bongmba, Ph.D., is the Harry and Hazel Chair in Christian Theology and Professor of Religion at Rice University. Bongmba, a native of Cameroon, combines his teaching of African religions and his research in theology and philosophy of religion working with African philosophical ideas and Continental philosophy. Professor Bongmba is the president of the African Association for the Study of Religion (2010–2015), managing editor at Religious Studies Reviews, and editor of The Routledge Companion to Christianity in Africa, and The Wiley Blackwell Companion to African Religions. Professor Bongmba has authored: *African Witchcraft and Otherness: A Philosophical and Theological Critique of Intersubjective Relations; The Dialectics of Transformation in Africa* (winner of the 2007 Franz Fanon Prize for Outstanding Work in Caribbean Thought); and *Facing a Pandemic: The African Church and the Crisis of AIDS.*